The

Straight

Skinny

Honest talk about dieting without the hype and political correctness

William W. "Skip" Simonds

with Wickham B. Simonds, M.D.

ISBN: 9781980971313

ACKNOWLEDGEMENTS

We are indebted to Eric Westman, M.D. whose knowledge and understanding of the entire subject matter was both essential and inspiring. We are also greatly appreciative of Stephanie Lugg and her editorial skill and attention to detail that made us look good!

CONTENTS

PREFACE

My nephew, Wickham Bryant Simonds, saved my life.

Really.

But I'm getting ahead of myself.

Wickham began his career as a medic in the US Army, serving in Korea. Upon completing his enlistment, he attended college and medical school to obtain his M.D. and began his professional work as an Emergency Room physician, the logical extension of his desire to help people that began as a medic. As Dr. Simonds' experience developed, he realized that as an ER physician he was too often treating the results of poor choices people were making in the personal lives, rather than having the ability to affect those choices.

Since, from his perspective, most of the trauma he dealt with in the ER was either the direct result of or complicated significantly by conditions of obesity, Dr. Simonds decided to take the next logical step in his career as he opened the first physician centered weight loss practice in western North Carolina. Thus began his attempt to affect his clients health at the source, through effective weight management.

That's where I came into the picture. I'm a consultant and Dr. Simonds was in need of some business consulting, so he called on me. At the conclusion of one of our consultations, Dr. Simonds looked at me and said something so simple yet so profound, that it literally changed my life.

"Uncle Skip, I love you, and I don't want you to die. But if you don't lose some weight, you're going to, and too soon as far as

I'm concerned. I'd like to have you around for a long time yet."

I could not ignore that plea. We talked about strategies, basically what we are going to share with you in this short book, and I started that night.

I was 65 years old, 5' 11" tall, and weighed over 210 pounds (I say "over" because I don't know exactly how much I weighed and was into my new lifestyle for several days before I weighed in). My BMI (Body Mass Index - an imperfect but nonetheless important measure of obesity) was borderline "morbid obesity". I was a severe medical condition waiting to happen. I knew it. He knew it. Everyone knew it. But he had the courage to call me out on it.

Dr. Simonds is a man of strong feelings. If you ever meet him, one thing you get is that he doesn't waffle. If he knows, he'll tell you. If he doesn't know, he won't guess. He'll study and investigate and find out. He doesn't have opinions, he has views that are typically born out of life experience, training, and dogged determination.

What he is going to share with you is that kind of stuff. He's going to say in this book the same thing he would say to you if you were sitting in his office. He's going to tell you the truth, insofar as he knows it. And he's not going to pull any punches to make sure he doesn't offend anyone. He's just going to tell it straight.

In the military, the truth is often called "skinny". "Straight skinny" is the purest and most unadulterated truth possible. That's why we're calling this book, "The Straight Skinny."

William W. "Skip" Simonds
The Coast of Maine
May 2018

1

DIET CHOICES
They Aren't Unlimited

The number of diets out there is legion. Staggering. Bewildering. There are so many, no one can possibly know them all, and no one can possibly be expected to understand which one will actually work for them.

Go to the bookstore or an online book seller and go to the diet section and check. I just plugged in the word "diet" to Amazon's search function and limited the results to "books". I got 117,800 hits.

Let me simplify life for you. There are only two choices when it comes to diets for the purposes of losing weight, and that's because your body isn't unlimited in the way it responds to the food you eat. Here are your choices:

1. Restricted Calorie Diets - Most are Low-Fat. Common examples would be Calorie Counting and Weight Watchers. These are essentially high carb diets with some protein and very little fat. This category also includes Low Fat Diets - based on the idea that if you're fat, you should eat less fat. This approach results in eating a diet that is high in carbohydrates and some protein, but because fats are relatively high in calories, eliminating it makes this a specific variation (and a very popular one) of a restricted calorie diet.

2. Low Carbohydrate Diets - This diet is a high fat diet that incorporates moderate protein intake and employs intense carbohydrate restriction. Your body burns your own fat stores as its energy source which can produce weight loss. The most well known example of this type of diet is the Atkins Diet.

A word about a word: diet

Technically diet is "the sum total of all food consumed by an individual", i.e. what you eat. But more often it is "a temporary eating regimen designed to lose a certain amount of weight." If that's what you are interested in, then forget it. You can diet. You'll lose weight. And then you'll gain it all back again, plus some more. Better you don't diet in the first place. Seriously. Put this book away and go find a cookbook. This book is about CHANGING WHAT YOU EAT for the rest of your life, not about "DOING A DIET PLAN."

All the multitude of diets you have heard of (and the 117,800 on Amazon) fit into one of these two categories. They are variations on a theme, for sure, but they work (if they work) because they fall into one of these categories because your body can only do so much in terms of digesting, using, and eliminating food.

The key (and we mean this literally - what you are about to read is The Key) to all dieting is understanding how your body handles the food you eat. **After all, it isn't food that makes you lose or gain weight; it is what your body does or doesn't do with the food you eat.**

Let's take this just a tad further. Your body's inability to properly handle the food you eat can create actual injury to your system which is where a lot of weight gain comes from. The type of food you eat and the amount of food you eat can actually damage the weight control center of the brain making it increasingly difficult to lose weight and keep weight off once it is lost.

So what really drives weight loss is understanding how your body handles food and adjusting your food intake accordingly. What we need to do is not "go on a diet", but rather "change our diet". When we understand how our bodies handle the food we eat, it is incumbent on us to adjust our eating habits accordingly.

So in this book, when we talk about diets, we are talking about everything you eat from now on...not some specialized meal plan that you're going to do for the next 8 weeks until you reach your weight loss goal.

Let me say this a slightly different way: your present diet got you into the place where you are seriously reading this book. Unless that diet changes, permanently, you are not going to change your weight or

Dieting: food insanity

If the definition of insanity is doing the same thing repeatedly but expecting a different outcome, then for most folks, dieting is insanity. No one seriously diets to lose weight for a short period and then expects to regain that weight. But they do. And then they "diet" again. Insanity.

health over the long term for the better. Do what you want "to lose weight", but if you don't change what you eat permanently, so that it works with your body's own biology, you are logically doomed to find yourself right back here reading this paragraph again. It may take a month, a year, or a decade; but you'll be back here again.

I suspect that for some of you reading this, this isn't your first rodeo. You've "dieted" before. So let's make this your last "diet" by changing what you eat!

If desire to change were the true means to change, we'd all be changed. If desire to lose weight through better eating (whatever that is) were the key, we'd all have lost weight and kept it off.

I'm not telling you to "get hot" or "get fired up" or "come to Jesus". Why? Because that doesn't work in the long run. What you need is better information about your body and how it works so that you understand why the choices you make about food matter and what the impact of those choices are on you, short and long term.

In this book, we are going to strongly recommend a lifestyle change. Anything short of that is pointless. Temporary measures to achieve weight loss are just that, temporary. We see no value and actually a significant downside to simply losing weight for the short term only to gain it all back, plus a bit more. Not only is future weight loss more difficult, there are deleterious effects on your body and its metabolism.

That's because obesity is a disease. Don't get hung up on the word "obesity." We use it to indicate a weight that is excessive given your body and lifestyle. If you consider yourself "overweight",

What do you like to eat?

This sounds really basic (and to many dietitians, just plain wrong), but the right ongoing diet for you probably has more to do with what foods you like than with finding "the right food". After all, if you are going to make a lifestyle change, it's easier to maintain it if you actually like the food you are eating rather than eating foods you think you ought to like because they're "good for you."

recognize that whether your weight fits the technical definition of obesity or not, that is probably only a matter of pounds and time. The disease of obesity is at work in you.

Yes, we meant to say that. **Obesity is a disease. Your weight is a symptom of that disease, not the disease itself.** You can lose the weight, but until and unless you deal with the disease, the disease remains, lurking in the background, awaiting the opportunity to reassert itself.

What you eat can treat the disease or bring it on. That's why we are so serious about this topic.

It is important that you learn about your physiology and metabolism, and learn about how they work with the food you eat. The goal is to gain a better knowledge of the interaction of food with your body, and then make some life altering decisions. After that you can make an informed, knowledgeable decision with the long view in mind.

Our perspective, as you'll see, is skewed to the low carb, ketogenic end of the spectrum. For us, the science and clinical experience in treating thousands of obese patients validates that a ketogenic diet outperforms all others, has the best outcomes, the longest lasting results, requires the least energy to maintain it, and has the best long term health outcomes.

So let's get started. We will look at your body's physiology as it relates to obesity and eating. We will look at food types (there's simplicity there, too, believe it or not) and what each does in your body. And we will look at how you actually eat.

We promise you this will be simple, easy to understand, and straight forward. There are no food eating plans, no diet stages, no excess of rules and regulations. We are just going to point you in the right direction, equipped with the right information, and make you cognizant of the appropriate principles to make good, sound lifestyle choices.

2

FOOD TYPES
making good choices based on your body

In our goal to make and keep things simple, we'd like for you to get used to the idea that food is like diets: there are 1,000's of kinds of foods you can eat, but they all are primarily made up of three basic components (called macronutrients).

Proteins
Carbohydrates
Fats

Now this may seem like a great oversimplification, and to a professional dietitian, for example, it is. But when it comes to gaining or losing weight, your body doesn't care a lot about the finer points. It deals with foods based on the relative composition of these macronutrients.

Let's take the big three in order.

Proteins are the building blocks of life. Every cell in your body has proteins. Proteins are made up of chains of amino acids and your body uses those amino acids (breaks them down, recombines them, rearranges them) for the maintenance of cells and for cell growth.

Everyone needs protein in their diet; that is not questioned. However, the consensus is that protein is so readily available in most diets that people rarely need to supplement their diet with additional protein.

Can you eat too much protein? Yes. In that you can eat too much anything, you certainly can. Is that all that likely to happen in most diets? Not really, but in some diets that reduce carbohydrates or fats, you may want to be aware of the amount of protein you are eating because if

6

Food Nutrition Labels
Those nutrition labels
haven't always been
around. They were
legislated in 1990 by the
Nutrition and Education
Labeling Act passed by
Congress. It became
standardized a year later.
These labels were
developed, like most
legislation, with the help of
"special interests". So bear
that in mind as you read
them.

you're not eating carbs or fat, you'll be eating a lot of protein. But even that isn't a real health risk unless you have diagnosed renal issues.

While there is nothing that suggests there are harmful ramifications of eating too much protein, if you are eating more than your body can digest, you'll gain weight. That's not good, obviously, especially since the point here is that you want to lose weight.

So how much protein is enough? Many experts suggest that 0.8 grams of protein per kilogram of weight is the minimum. So for a 150 pound person that would be 55 grams per day. For reference, that is about the size of a normal chicken breast. And considering that you'll be getting protein from lots of other things during the day, that's not a lot.

That's why the experts say that normally people do not need to supplement their normal food intake with additional protein.

OK. Let's talk carbs.

For a moment, if possible, forget everything you think you know about carbohydrates. Other than fats, I don't think there has been a food type that has more misinformation associated with it. Everyone, it seems, has something to say about carbs and, unfortunately, too much of it is uninformed. So let's just cut through all of that for a moment if we could, please.

Carbs are neither good nor bad. They are just, well, carbs. Carbohydrates are organic compounds in food that are most often found as sugars and starches, but they can also include fiber/cellulose.

The body typically breaks down the non-fiber carbs (if it can) into energy.

There are many different types of carbohydrates, and no doubt you've heard

There are two types of
fibers, soluble and
insoluble. One dissolves in
liquid (water), the other
doesn't. The insoluble kind
is the kind of fiber that
keeps you "moving" and
has no calories. The
soluble kind is treated by
the body just like
carbohydrates at 4 calories
per gram.

It's true both will help you
lose weight but for
different reasons. The
insoluble fills you up and
reduces your hunger,
thereby taking the place in
your diet of other foods
that have calories.

The soluble also
contributes to making you
feel full, but still adds
calories to you. However,
it may keep you from
eating more calories than
you would without it.

the good, the bad, and the ugly about each. For our purposes, the only real major difference we are concerned about is fiber carbohydrates. These can be separated out from all other carbohydrates (or not counted as carbs). Every other form of carbohydrate can be lumped together under the general rubric of "carbs." (See the sidebar for some critical information on fiber)

Now if we ask the same question about carbohydrates that we asked about protein - how much does a person need - the answer we get is going to be terribly different depending on who we ask. And then those answers are going to vary greatly depending on what kind of carbs (fiber versus non-fiber) we are talking about. This is where it all gets very confusing.

It is important to understand that fiber is NOT a macronutrient. It really has no food value to you. Fiber is just one of several strategies for keeping your body "regular" by moving food through your system.

How much fiber do we need to accomplish that? What that number is varies from person to person and with their diets. However, it is almost universally agreed that the number needs to be north of 20 grams per day.

It's all the rest of the types of carbs other than fiber about which there is such a difference of opinion. But as a general rule of thumb, the number of grams of carbohydrates you need is less important than getting the number of calories you need in your diet.

So as an example, if you know that you need 60 grams of protein and at least 20 grams of fiber, that will mean you've eaten about 240 calories (all from the protein because fiber passes through your system

Measuring Food

There are two major ways to think about "how much" as it applies to food. One way is by weight, and most typically, is expressed in grams. One gram is a little more than 3/100 of an ounce. It takes almost 29 grams to make an ounce. So a gram is s-m-a-l-l.

The other way to think of food is by calories. Calories are a unit of energy. As you can imagine some foods are better at delivering energy than others...they have more calories by weight.

In general, carbohydrates and proteins deliver 4 calories per gram of food. Fat delivers 9 calories per gram of food.

without a caloric impact). So if you need 1400 calories to sustain your activity level, that means you can eat the balance in non-fiber carbohydrates (forgetting fat for the moment).

Like protein, most people do not need any type of supplement for getting enough non-fiber carbohydrates. Given that sugars, both natural and refined, are virtually 100% carbohydrates, on that level alone, we get plenty.

Add in the fact that starches (potatoes, grains, root vegetables) are carbohydrate rich, and you can see that the average person has no shortage of carbs in his or her diet.

The main challenge with non-fiber carbohydrates is to not eat too many "cheap" carbs, those rich in refined sugar (think "Twinkie" end of the spectrum) because they pour on the calories with no real beneficial impact to the body.

But how many grams of carbohydrates do you NEED? That's a great question and one that is being hotly debated by various dietary authorities. The answer, which is so simple for protein and fiber, is very much more complicated for non-fiber carbs. However, we are going to make it simple for you to understand.

There is universal agreement that there are essential proteins (amino acids) and essential fats. These are different from other proteins and fats in that research has shown that your body needs them for life. However, your body does not manufacture them, so you must get them from what you eat. That's why they are called "essential".

However, it is important to note that there are NO essential carbohydrates.

In Chapter 3 we are going to talk about how your body actually handles the food you eat. And we're going to find that what

Cell "fat"

If you remember your 10th grade anatomy course, you may recall that the human body is made up of systems, and that each system is made up of organs, and each organ is made up of cells.

Well, let's take it one step further, each cell is made up of a bunch of components, but one of the most prevalent is the cell wall, that thing that holds the cell together. It is made up of molecules of lipids.

Lipids are cool. They are also a fat.

kinds of food you eat, and the amounts of each you eat, to a great extent determines how your body handles that food.

So hang in there. Chapter 3 is coming up.

Fat.

Let's talk about fat.

Like protein and carbs, fat is an energy source, but it also provides a structural component for the body.

Similar to carbohydrates, the body can use fat for energy right away by converting it into an energy source, albeit by a different process (and that will be important to know when we get to Chapter 3).

Fat can also be stored for use as an energy source later, and it is used especially when the body is under stress.

Fat is also a source of lipids which are molecules that are the building blocks of cell walls.

So are we concerned about the types of fat we eat? From a health perspective, yes. But from a weight loss perspective, no. There are a ton of books and articles out there about the various of types of fats and the health ramifications of each, and we recommend that you don't worry about familiarizing yourself with them. Why? Because when you are eating properly, the differences may largely become irrelevant.

For now we are going to lump all those types of fats together because, by and large, the body tends to handle them all the same way from a digestion, weight gain/loss, perspective. The only exception is trans-fats, which if you'll eat properly, as we'll discuss, will not be a problem.

So, how much fat should I be getting in my diet?

When most diet gurus talk about fats in the daily diet they tend to talk in terms of

Fat is ubiquitous
If you've ever been on a low fat diet, you know that fat is a huge part of the civilized world's diet. It is seen overtly in fried foods, salad dressings, condiments, and deserts. But it is also hidden in the formulas of lots of foods you don't think of as fat carriers.

And just because something says it is low fat, doesn't mean it is actually low fat. It only means it is low fat relative to it's "regular" fat cousins.

an upper limit. The assumption is that fats are "dense" foods (they are - remember a gram of fat has 225% of the calories of a gram protein or carbohydrates) and so overeating fat is of greater concern than under eating. That's why you don't generally see "fat supplements" for sale.

The conventional wisdom says to limit your fat intake to 20% to 35% of your daily caloric intake. So, by example, if you typically are eating 1,400 calories a day, that means you will want to eat no more than 280 to 490 calories of fat.

Doing the math, that means that your daily intake of fat should be no more than somewhere between 31 to 54 grams of fat. Er... that's 1-2 ounces of fat. Eat a dark chocolate bar. That's your fat for the entire day. Everything else you eat must be fat free.

That includes the French fries, the 1/2 scoop of vanilla ice cream, the half & half in your coffee, the mayo on your turkey breast sandwich... You get where I'm going with this. You can scarf up your entire day's allotment of fat without blinking.

That's the conventional wisdom, and we aren't arguing with that. But it assumes a number of things, none the least of which is that you are getting most of your calories from carbs and some from proteins.

And that is a great segue to Chapter 3, because as you'll see, we do take on the conventional wisdom and question the assumptions associated with it.

But to do that you have to understand how your body handles all these macronutrients we've been talking about.

3

YOUR BODY
and its metabolic pathways

Let's forget about diets and dieting for a moment and talk about how your body works when it comes to food. We're going to be a little over simplistic here, but this is one of those subjects where you can get really bogged down in the detail.

Your body is either going to digest carbs and store fat, or digest fat and store carbs.

It is really that simple. Seriously.

Which it does depends almost entirely on the type and quantity of foods you eat. But fundamentally that is all your body is capable of: digesting carbs or fat, one or the other, not both at the same time...except if you are on a very, very low calorie diet combined with a very rigorous exercise program where your caloric needs far outstrip the caloric supply of the food you eat.

We hate caveats like that, but we have to in include it because it's true. However, it doesn't come into play here because we are talking about a lifestyle change, not a short term diet to lose weight. A stringent calorie restricted diet combined with a high energy exercise regimen is a short term strategy, typically as part of a high performance training program...or a "Biggest Loser" reality TV show. And that's just not what we're talking about here. A long term program that you have a prayer of maintaing is going to be one that either draws on carb or fat digestion, even if it is a calorie counting diet.

So for regular folks like you and me, that dictum: either digest carbs/store fat or digest fat/store carbs is the bottom line.

12

Metabolic Pathways for
Dummies
The whole deal on what
your body does with the
food you eat has to do
with creating energy
sources for the individual
cells in your body (of which
you have a little over 37
trillion - that's 37 with 12,
count 'em, 12 zeros!). And
everyone of those little
guys is dependent on the
food you eat to deliver the
energy source it needs to
do the work it is supposed
to do. So your body has a
couple of different
"pathways" to break down
your food which it can use
depending on the food
you're eating.

That's pretty cool when
you think about it. Much
like a computer with the
ability to run both an Apple
and a Windows operating
system, your body has a
"dual operating system" to
maximize the energy
production for your cells.

Your body takes the food that you eat, and starting with chewing and adding saliva, begins a process of breaking it down into useable components for energy, growth, and maintenance. Your body can't use pasta, but it can use the carbohydrates, protein, and fat that make it up.

You don't need to have a course in anatomy and physiology to understand this. It is fundamentally pretty simple how the body deals with foods. Your whole digestive system is designed to break the food you eat down into its constituent parts (mainly those macronutrients we talked about in Chapter 2) in a succession of processes that starts with chewing in your mouth and ends with absorption in your intestines.

It really doesn't matter what kind of food you eat. Whatever you eat goes through that breakdown process to get it into usable form for your body.

What is critical though is what your body does with those macronutrients once they've been liberated in a useable form.

Essentially your body has two major and pretty different metabolic processes or states to deal with those macronutrients once they are ready for your body to use. Digestion gets them ready for use. Metabolism then actually uses them.

The two metabolic processes are a glycolytic and a ketotic state, and they are mutually exclusive in that only one can be the dominant state at any one time. So your body either does primarily one or the other. And which one is dominant depends almost entirely on what the predominant macronutrients are that you eat.

Actually, we can put an even finer point on that last sentence. Your body is very sensitive to non-fiber carbohydrates and

The Caveman Theory
Some unscientific but interesting articles suggest the reason the human body has two metabolic pathways rather than just one is due to evolutionary pressure.

As the theory goes, cavemen were alternatively "gatherers" during part of the year when plants and fruits were plentiful and "hunters" during that part of the year when plant based food was not readily available.

This would mean that part of the year they'd eat a diet rich in carbs and low in fat; and part of the year the opposite. During the growing season, they'd digest carbs and store what little fat they ate for the future through glycolysis. During hunting season, they'd start digesting the fat they'd stored and were eating and store what few carbs they'd eat through ketosis.

Of course no one knows how accurate the theory is, but it does make sense.

fat, less so about protein, and not much at all about fiber. If you eat more than a certain amount of non-fiber carbohydrates per day, your body "defaults" to utilizing the glycolytic state as its main energy production process.

However, if you eat less than that amount and replace those carbs with fat calories, your body will "switch over" to the ketotic state for as long as you maintain that higher fat to non-fiber carbohydrate ratio. (Don't worry. We'll get more specific in a bit. Right now we just want you to understand the basic concepts of the two metabolic states.)

So what are these two pathways and how do they differ?

Again, in an effort to keep this very simple, when your body is utilizing glycolysis, you are digesting carbohydrates for present energy demands and storing fat for future energy needs.

When your body is in a ketotic state, the opposite occurs. Your body is digesting fat for it's energy demands and storing carbohydrates for reserves for the future.

Because our "natural" diet in most of the civilized world is dominated by carbohydrates, our bodies continually use the glycolytic process to generate energy since our daily intake of carbs is almost always higher than the "tipping point" below which the ketotic state could kick in and the glycolytic state would tone down.

And because there is a societal preference, for whatever reason, for carbohydrate dominated food intake, there is very little talk about the ketotic state because it does not occur "naturally" in societies that eat mostly carbs.

In fact, most of what you've probably heard about the ketotic state (often called ketosis) is bad, largely due to its association

Caveman Part 2
Why is losing weight so much harder and takes so much longer than gaining weight?

Well, again evolutionary theory suggests (but doesn't prove) a theory.

When you overeat, the food you don't use for energy or eliminate gets stored on your body for future energy needs. In evolutionary terms, your body is always assuming there is going to be a future time where food for energy is scarce, so like the old saying, "Get all you can, and can all you get!", it rather quickly and efficiently stores the excess as body fat/mass.

But when you do hit "the famine", your body continues to be conservative and only withdraws from "reserves" (a nice way of saying fat) exactly what it needs, and hoards the rest.

Hence, easy on, hard off.

with diabetes. When we are referring to a ketotic state, we are talking about "nutritional ketosis" and it is safe and promotes excellent health as it is a natural digestive process in your body. Diabetics can get "keto-acidosis" (or DKA) which is a totally different thing. It is dangerous and potentially fatal. It is important to note that DKA is not in any way brought on by eating a low carb diet. Because the names sound somewhat similar, people often think these are the same thing. They are not.

But it is important to note that the ketotic state is a normal metabolic state that the healthy body is capable of initiating and sustaining. In our society many people are never in the ketotic state and it remains a "backup" state for energy generation, i.e. to digest diets rich in fats and low in carbohydrates.

Let's say it straight up: to be in a ketotic state as a response to the ratio of fats to carbohydrates you are eating is not unhealthy. It is normal. Your body is designed to do that.

But what about protein, you ask? Proteins fall into an "either/or" category. And I apologize in advance, but this is a little complicated. What happens to protein in your body is dependent on a couple of things.

Protein has its own metabolic pathway if you will. Our bodies need a certain amount of protein to maintain our lean body mass (which is defined as everything that makes up our body that isn't fat). How many grams of protein that is tends to be a "sliding scale" which depends on your lean body mass. The accepted level of protein is defined as 0.6-1.0 gram of protein per pound of lean body mass. At this level, your body uses that protein to repair and build lean body mass. Less than

The "Fat/Carb" Nexus
From the perspective of your metabolic pathways, fats and carbohydrates are almost like enemies. You're always digesting one and storing the other as fat/mass on your body.

Yuck.

But when they are in combination (and they are in combination a lot) the combination reinforces itself. The carbs, especially sugar carbs, gives you that great energy rush. And the fat is that really satisfying texture and taste that makes you feel full and not hungry anymore.

So over the years, like Pavlov and his dogs, we've reinforced the idea of the combination of the two macronutrients as "pleasurable".

We even call them "guilty pleasures."

this, and the body uses the protein you eat and then uses the protein stored in your body to make up the difference for your body's lean mass needs. Obviously, that's not ideal and should be avoided. You want to maintain and even increase lean body mass, not deplete it.

When you eat more than 1.0 gram of protein per pound of lean body mass per day, a significant portion is converted into glucose which your body responds to as though you were eating carbohydrates. So you could be on a low carbohydrate diet, but if you are eating too much protein, it is as though you are not.

Thus, eating more protein will cause your body to increase insulin production, restart the glycolytic process, and overshadow the ketotic process again. In short, it will be as though you were eating more carbs.

Often times people who are on a "low carb" diet try to help that diet along by eating a "low fat" form of that diet: eating low carbs and low fat. Of course that means you are eating a "high protein" diet because your calories have to come from somewhere.

You may have noticed in Chapter 1, we didn't include "high protein" as one of the basic types of diets to lose weight. That's because as you can see, practically your body doesn't really differentiate between high protein or high carb. They both are treated like a "low fat" diet.

So if you are in a ketotic state and eat "high protein, low fat", you will not be in that state for long.

Perhaps this is a good time to talk about how your body switches from a glycolytic state to a ketotic one and back again. I know it sounds like it can be almost automatic and immediate, but it isn't.

To the "pros" reading this: If you are a doc or a dietary specialist, we know we have way over simplified the biology here. But we have a good reason. We didn't write this book for you.

We wrote it for regular, everyday folks who don't have medical degrees and who haven't studied advance topics in diet, chemistry, and physiology. If we satisfied your need for precision, we would have left the folks we are trying to help even more confused and befuddled than they already are.

If you, the professional, want more information about this part of the discussion, we'd recommend you get a copy of "The Art and Science of Low Carbohydrate Living" by Volek & Phinney (2011). That should help bridge the gap for you between what we've written here for the lay person and what you as a professional need.

Have you ever noticed how easy it is to gain weight but how hard it is to actually lose weight? Well, the process of transitioning from one metabolic pathway to another is sort of like that.

As a general rule it is much harder to go from a glycolytic state to a ketotic one than it is to go the opposite direction. Conventional wisdom suggests it takes about two weeks for the average person to go from a glycolytic state to a ketotic one and get his or her body firmly established in that pathway.

We think that is probably a tad overly conservative, but it definitely takes several days of some pretty significant diet change to make it happen.

But going the opposite direction, from a ketotic state back to a glycolytic one can be accomplished in a day, perhaps even in hours, in some cases even with just one meal.

Seriously? Yes, seriously.

The reason is because, in really unscientific terms, your body uses your insulin to support glycolysis. If insulin is present in sufficient quantities in your body, you are in the glycolytic state. If insulin is not present in sufficient quantities, then your body is in a ketotic state. So insulin is the trigger.

The process of going from a glycolytic state to a ketotic one takes time because you have to "quiet" your system down and get your insulin below a level where it "triggers" glycolysis. Insulin, even when production is slowed way down, doesn't just instantly disappear from your system. It takes time.

However, going the opposite direction, from a ketotic state to a glycolytic one, your body can produce insulin literally within an hour or two, and boom, the glycolytic state returns to dominance.

And once that happens, you're back to at least several days of transition to return to ketosis, if that's what you want to do. If you have been in the ketotic state solidly for more than a couple of weeks, it won't take as much time to get back to it, but it will still take a period of time measured in days. And if you haven't been "adapted" for that long, you could be looking at up to two weeks.

OK, so let's think about this from a weight perspective since that's what this book is all about.

An overly simplistic way of putting this is that our body is always, whether you are in a glycolytic or ketotic state, primarily digesting one of the macronutrients and storing a second. You are either primarily digesting carbs and storing fat or digesting fat and storing carbs.

So, it follows that regardless of which metabolic pathway you are in, the worst combination of foods you can eat if you want to lose weight or maintain weight loss is carbohydrates with fat. No matter what your metabolic pathway is, that food is going to have some element that is going to get stored as body fat/mass.

4

SEE SAW

more detail than you probably wanted to know on how your body handles food

In dealing with the metabolic states in this book we have used the term "pathways" on occasion. That word is a picture word and we used it on purpose so that you would understand that these "states" are not just static, but dynamic with cascading effects that lead to different outcomes.

It also played strongly into helping you to see and become confident in the idea that you can pick the pathway you want your body to "walk" in. Remember from Chapter 1 we told you that "...it isn't food that makes you fat. It is what your body does with the food you eat that makes you fat." Choosing the right pathway is critical to losing weight and maintaining that weight loss.

However, the problem with the "pathway" analogy is that while it is a great differentiator, it is not completely accurate with how your body actually operates.

As you now know, your body has two metabolic states: glycotic and ketotic. Your body has both pathways operating at the same time. One is dominant and one is not. But you are never completely in one and not the other. Both are present all the time.

So our analogy of pathways or states has this flaw: it too easily suggests an either/or situation, and that is not how your body works.

Your body is very complex and responds to the food you eat in complex ways. However, the "triggers" that determine how the two fundamental complex processes are going to work at any time are incredibly simple.

In a verbal nutshell it works like this.

Your body has a three stage energy usage and storage system. One is immediate, one is intermediate, and one is long term. The immediate one is for immediate energy needs for your body and its individual cells. It's called glucose and it is in your blood all the time. For most folks it's present at the level of up to 1 gram per liter of blood. You have somewhere between 5 and 7 liters of blood, so your immediate energy needs equate to a really, really small amount of blood sugar...up to 5 to 7 grams. And, man, that is small. It is about the size of a teaspoon of sugar or a little less. Think about it. That's all the sugar your body says it needs for its immediate energy needs.

The intermediate storage is called your glycogen stores, and they are kept in the liver and muscles. The stores are readily converted into glucose, but are not present in the circulation until needed. When your immediate needs deplete the glucose level in your blood, your body converts the glycogen stores into glucose to replenish it.

The long term storage is body fat. And when your glycogen stores are depleted your body has two options. First, if you are eating carbohydrates, it will convert the carbs into glycogen stores, or use any excess protein you are eating as a source of glucose. Or if you are not eating carbs, your body will start to convert the fat into ketones which are interchangeable with glucose in that your body's energy needs can be met by ketones just like they are met from glucose.

Now this is the important part. Insulin is the key factor in determining whether your body is in a glycolytic state or a state of ketosis. The amount of insulin in your body is determined by the carbohydrates you eat. The more you eat, the more insulin your body produces. The fewer carbohydrates you eat, the less insulin your body produces. And if you eat below a certain level of carbohydrates, your body produces a level of insulin that is functionally invisible to your body.

Ketones are in your body all the time, but if you are eating enough carbohydrates to supply all your energy needs, your body doesn't burn a lot of fat and therefore only generates a small amount of ketones. Insulin is the fat storage hormone. When the insulin level is elevated it signals the body to store and hold on to fat rather than to release fat and burn it. This higher insulin level is why excess carbohydrate intake (beyond your body's immediate and intermediate needs) is converted into fat for long term storage.

You see where we are going with this, right?

The only way you are going to lose body fat and maintain that weight loss is to start burning that stored body fat and turning it into energy. But since that is the last process in the three process link, that isn't going to happen until you are using more glucose and glycogen than can be produced by the carbohydrates you eat.

Read that last sentence again. It is important.

The presence of carbohydrates in your system stimulates insulin production. Insulin operates to create stores of energy, intermediate and long term, for all the extra carbs you eat over and above what you need.

And you don't need a lot. That fact that you have less than 1 teaspoon of "sugar" in your blood at any given time tells you that your energy demands are way less than you probably thought.

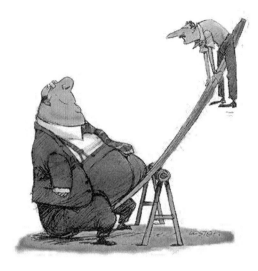

So when you eat a carb laden dinner of pasta, with 40 grams of carbohydrates per 1 cup serving, you are eating 8X your body's immediate energy needs! And the more carbs you eat, the more insulin is produced because there is more energy to be managed and stored.

But when you eat fewer carbs, less insulin is produced, so less energy needs to be stored. So this whole deal really is controlled by the number of carbs you eat.

Actually, the ketotic state is present all along, but is so overshadowed by the carbs you eat that it rarely does more than just a little bit of work and what little it takes out of fat stores is more than replaced by the carbs being converted into fat.

So here's an analogy to help you grasp this. Think of your metabolic states like a see-saw with two little kids on one side (Carbs and Insulin) and one big kid on the other side (Ketones). The more carbs you eat the bigger the Carb kid gets, and the bigger the Carb kid gets, the bigger the Insulin kid gets. And when those two are big enough, the teeter-totter puts them both on the ground with Ketone kid stuck in the air.

You can't make Ketone kid bigger. But you can eat fewer carbs which will make Carb kid and Insulin kid smaller. Eventually, if you eat few enough carbs, Ketone kid will be sitting firmly on the ground, in complete control.

At that point, Ketone kid is digesting your fat faster than your body can replenish it.

So with that analogy in your head, realize two very, very significant things.

First, only the number of carbs you eat can impact which side of the teeter-totter is on the ground. It doesn't matter how much fat you eat or don't eat. The see-saw stays weighted in favor of Carb and Insulin, and with your body's energy needs being so low, you are really fighting against yourself to lose weight. Ouch.

Second, and we think this is the money shot if you will, the ketotic state does not require a counterpart to insulin in order to kick in. It automatically kicks in anytime the insulin levels go down and stay down below a certain point. What that means is (and here it is - the payoff) that the ketotic state is your body's basic, fundamental, default state; not the glycolytic state. The glycolytic state requires insulin to operate. We believe that the glycolytic state was designed by evolution to be a temporary state - a very small energy store. The body is designed to function primarily in a ketotic state supplemented as necessary by glycolysis and insulin (i.e. when only carbs are available).

So remember that teeter-totter and realize it is you who controls that balance based on what types of food you choose to eat.

5

CHOOSING A LIFESTYLE
moving forward with a plan

Elsewhere we've mentioned that oft used definition of insanity: "doing the same thing over and over again but expecting different results." That's kind of where you are right now.

You're reading this book, so clearly you're not happy with the previous results of the choices you've made.

You've read a straightforward account in the previous three chapters about what your body does with the different types of foods you eat.

You've learned that your body has different ways to handle different foods.

And you've learned that when it comes to losing weight, in spite of what it looks like, you've really only got two fundamental choices.

So the question is: do you want to go on a diet (something you've done before, probably repeatedly, that's led you to right here)? Or do you want to change your diet (and therefore adopt a new nutritional lifestyle)?

If you want to go on a diet and lose a few pounds, stop reading now. Seriously. Stop. Put this book down. We have no further information or wisdom for you. We're neither mad at or disappointed in you. It's your choice. We'll be right here if you decide to come back.

But....

If you want to change your diet and lifestyle, then stick with us for at least the rest of this chapter. We'd like to help you make that decision in a way that will maximize your chances for true, life long change.

Finding the Path

"If you learn only methods, you'll be tied to your methods, but if you learn principles you can devise your own methods."
— Ralph Waldo Emerson

"Always bear in mind that our own resolution to succeed is more important than any other one thing."
— Abraham Lincoln

We want to remind you of what you read back in Chapter 1:

There are only two choices when it comes to diets, and that's because your body isn't unlimited in the way it responds to the food you eat. Here are your choices:

1. Restricted Calorie Diets - Most are Low-Fat. Common examples would be Calorie Counting and Weight Watchers. These are essentially high carb diets with some protein and very little fat.

2. Low Carbohydrate Diets - This diet is a high fat diet that incorporates moderate protein intake and employs intense carbohydrate restriction. Your body burns your own fat stores as its energy source which can produce weight loss. The most well known example of this type of diet is the Atkins Diet.

All the multitude of diets you have heard of (and the 117,800 we found on Amazon) fit into one of these two categories. They are variations on a theme, for sure, but they work (if they work) because they fall into one of these categories because your body can only do so much in terms of digesting, using, and eliminating food.

Now, combine that with the thought we're trying to drive home that if you want to change your body permanently, you need to change your diet lifestyle. On which of the two "principles" (to quote Emerson) do you want to base the "methods" of your life?

For Dr. Simonds and myself, the answer was obvious and immediate. We have chosen the Low Carbohydrate lifestyle. But that's our choice, not necessarily yours. As we've indicated before, we think it is the best, most healthy, easiest to maintain; but then again, if you can't do it, none of that

The Lifestyle Conundrum
It almost doesn't matter which of the diet lifestyles is "better for you." If you can't stay on it, even the best one isn't the best one for you. The best one for you is the one you can maintain.

matters. The main benefit of any change in diet has to be a healthier you. If a high fat, low carb diet is impossible for you to maintain, the health benefits of eating that way don't matter because, for you, they're unattainable.

So by default, your only other choice is a low calorie (and therefore low fat) lifestyle.

Let's review the advantages and risks of a low calorie low fat regimen. The following is reproduced from The Obesity Algorithm®, ©2018 Obesity Medicine Association.

First, let's look at the low calorie diet. This diet restricts daily caloric intake to fewer calories than your level of activities is currently burning, often 1000-1200 calories per day or less.

Weight Loss
- Depending on the daily intake of calories, it can produce more rapid weight loss than standard carbohydrate and/or fat-restricted dietary intake.

Metabolic Effects
- Reduces fasting glucose and insulin levels
- Reduces triglyceride levels
- May modestly increase high-density lipoprotein cholesterol levels
- May modestly decrease low-density lipoprotein cholesterol
- Reduces blood pressure

Risks
- Fatigue, nausea, constipation, diarrhea, hair loss, and brittle nails

- Cold intolerance
- Dysmenorrhea
- Gallstones
- Kidney stones
- Gout

If insufficient mineral intake, then may predispose to:

- Palpitations and cardiac dysrhythmias
- Muscle cramps
- Possible increased risk of osteoporosis
- Tooth decay

Granted, a lot of these risks are only seen with extremely low calorie diets in the range of 800 kcal/day or less. However, they are potential risks of any low calorie diet and should be watched for.

The upside is, of course, a faster potential weight loss. The other major upside is that you do not have to worry about the types of foods you eat as much as simply making sure you meet the dietary requirements outlined in Chapter 2 and maintain a daily intake below the target number of calories.

And, in addition, if you factor in the number of calories you are burning, you can actually increase your daily caloric intake by the number of calories you burn with specific additional exercise.

This is a lifestyle of exercise and smaller, more carefully chosen portions.

Hey, we're not knocking it. It works. And it works for a lot of people. It worked for us, too, although neither of us was able to maintain our weight loss for the long term.

But many can and are. If that type of daily regimen appeals to you and you have confidence you can maintain it, you go!

Changing a lifestyle is like turning an ocean going freighter around...it is slow and requires a lot of room for adjustment

"The main thing is to keep the main thing the main thing."
        - Steven Covey

And we will be rooting for you.

Let's take a look at a low fat variation of a restricted calorie diet using data from the same presentation. A low fat diet is often described as one that limits the fat intake to 20-30% or less of daily caloric intake.

Weight Loss

• After six months, fat-restrictive, low-calorie nutritional intervention generally produces the same amount of weight loss compared to the "low-carb diet"

Metabolic Effects

• May reduce fasting glucose and insulin levels

• Modestly decreases low-density and high-density lipoprotein cholesterol levels

• May modestly reduce blood pressure

Risks

• Hunger control may present challenges, which may be mitigated with weight-management pharmacotherapy.

• If fat restriction results in a substantial increase in carbohydrate consumption, and if weight loss is not achieved, then an increase in carbohydrate dietary intake may contribute to hyperglycemia, hyperinsulinemia, hyper-triglyceridemia, and reduced levels of high-density lipoprotein cholesterol.

To us it is interesting that a low fat diet lists as one of its risks some of the things normally associated with eating too much fat: hyperglycemia and hypertriglyceridemia. It is also interesting that the diet does little to deal with hunger and that the only recourse may be to hunger reducing drugs.

What's it going to take?

"Success is the sum of small efforts repeated day in and day out."
- Robert Collier

Still, this is a diet we have both tried and had moderate weight loss success...myself probably more than Wickham. But both of us found the lifestyle almost impossible to maintain in today's real world. The dietary prevalence of the combination of fat and carbohydrates in so many popular, easily available, and seemingly unavoidable foods is difficult to work around.

Keep in mind, with a low fat diet, your body is storing whatever fat it takes in provided it is getting enough energy from the carbs you're eating. So the diet works because you're not giving it enough fat to store. That explains why this variation is less effective at weight loss than the low calorie diet...because it is so hard if not impossible, to get below that minimum level of fat in your daily food intake.

Nor do you want to, by the way. You'll always need to eat some fat to maintain the intake of essential fatty acids.

In summary, both of these diet choices are fine for a lifestyle as long as you understand the impacts and risks. Of course, you should talk all of this over with your personal physician before embarking on any significant dietary change. Our approach is that we recommend you educate yourself about diet choices, impacts, and risks and then you'll have a much better conversation with your doctor.

Often your doctor may have their own special diet or slant on diets. They are trained professionals whose goal is the healthiest you possible. We just recommend you remember that no diet is successful if it cannot be maintained regardless of the benefits of the diet.

Make sure your physician knows that you are not talking about a short term food intake change, but rather a long term lifestyle food choice.

Now about the low carb diet...

Obviously we are biased. We admit it. We think the combination of getting most of your calories from fat, the least from carbohydrates, and protein somewhere in between is the best for a variety of reasons. And we hope we've shown you in Chapters 2 through 4 that it can be as healthy (if not more healthy) as any other choice.

But let's see what that same presentation has to say about a low carb lifestyle:

Weight Loss

• May produce modestly greater weight loss compared to fat-restricted dietary intake for the first 6 months, wherein afterwards, the net weight loss may be similar to other calorie restricted nutritional interventions

• May assist in fewer food cravings

Metabolic Effects

• Reduces fasting glucose and insulin levels

• Reduces triglyceride levels

• Modestly increases high-density lipoprotein cholesterol levels

• May modestly increase low-density lipoprotein cholesterol levels

• The metabolic effects noted above may occur with or without weight loss

• May modestly reduce blood pressure

• In patients with epilepsy, ketogenic diets may reduce seizures

• Ketogenic diet may possibly improve diabetes mellitus complications (i.e., nephropathy)

Risks

Which diet lifestyle is right for me

Instead of starting with the risk and rewards, or with your gut feeling on which diet lifestyle appeals to you, try this:

Make a list of foods you absolutely love and would eat more of if you could.

Make a list of foods you cannot possibly do without.

Make a list of foods you can easily do without.

See which diet lifestyle fits the closest with your tastes.

In the long run it is, after all, your tastes in food that will the greatest single determiner of and longest lasting influence on your food choices.

Find the best of the three diet lifestyles that lets you eat the food you love, allows you to keep the foods you cannot do without, and doesn't force you to eat the foods you hate in order to work.

• May produce carbohydrate cravings within the first few days of implementation, which may be mitigated by artificial sweeteners or adding low-glycemic-index foods

The two things that jump right off the page at us is almost startling. First, eating a high fat, low carb diet actually reduces all the things that we've been taught a low fat diet is supposed to do.

Second, the only significant risk is not medical, but emotional…"carbohydrate cravings".

This is one of the great reasons why Dr. Simonds and I are so high on this particular diet. The risks are minimal and the results are essentially all the ones you want and that are motivating you to change your lifestyle in the first place.

But…

As we said before, the choice is yours. We're rooting for you no matter what choice you make. And the choice is yours, no matter what we or anyone else says.

If you do want to choose (or at least explore some more) the high fat, low carb lifestyle, keep reading. We're going to call it HFLC for ease from here on.

If you think either a low calorie or low fat lifestyle is for you, we thank you for sticking with us this far and we hope we've made you a smarter dieter.

6

HLFC
getting started

Once you decide to change your lifestyle you actually have to change your lifestyle. Bummer.

This is going to be a really short chapter because what you really have to do is, well, get started and then just do it.

Here are three quick steps to getting unstuck from your current food insanity.

1. Get to the point where you really believe that fat is NOT the enemy! In point of fact, it is your friend.

2. Make yourself very familiar with which foods are high in carbohydrates and which are low.

3. Determine you will be OK with the judgmental reactions of well meaning friends when they see how you're eating.

We threw a quote at you in the last chapter in the margin by Robert Collier, a positive thinking, self help guru from the 1930's. "Success is the sum of small efforts repeated day in and day out." Moving ahead with an HLFC lifestyle is just that: a day by day change in the way to think about and respond to food and hunger. It isn't as exciting as getting a new job or getting married or having a baby. Those are big things.

This is all about what you're going to put in your mouth when you get hungry and put down this book. It's that mundane. It isn't even about what you're going to do later today, tomorrow, or next week. It's like AA...one step at a time...just decide to eat responsibly for the very next thing you put in your mouth. And then the thing after that. And then the thing after that.

Problem Solving
Losing weight is like solving
any problem.

"There is a solution to
every human problem -
neat, plausible, and
wrong."
                    - H.L. Mencken

We posit there are only
three axioms to losing
weight on the HFLC diet
lifestyle. Compare that to
the dictums of almost any
other diet regimen. We
live by it and it works.

There was an old movie back in the 1980's about an inventor played by, I think, Billy Crystal. He was a sour puss at the beginning of the movie and he invented a talking scale that if you weighed too much, would announce your weight and give some unsolicited advice.

He sold a few but they were all returned because the scale was as caustic as he was. As he explained, "No one wants a scale that when you step on it says, 'Your weight is 275 pounds. If you put anything else in your mouth today, it should be the muzzle of a loaded gun'."

The joke was funny but the point is real although not as the fictional inventor intended. Literally with every bite of food you select, you are choosing to put either something good or something bad in your mouth. Choose bites of food that will help you and move you to a more healthy weight and body function. Don't choose food which does not, no matter how good you think it tastes.

The goal of the HFLC lifestyle is to get into and stay in ketosis. This will happen automatically based on the proportion of fat, protein, and carbohydrates you eat. This will not happen immediately as it takes, on average, about two weeks to reduce insulin levels to the point where your body's ketotic track will kick in and take over. [If it has been a while since you read Chapter 4, we recommend you stop right now and go back and review it.]

With the HFLC lifestyle, there is no caloric maximum or minimum. There is only the ratio of fat to protein to carbs. Mind blowing, we know.

The target for an HFLC lifestyle is very simple:
    1.   **Calories:**   **60-70%** of your

Do not weigh every day. We recommend once a week at the same point of your day each week. For me, I weigh every Monday morning after I get up, after I take care of business in the bathroom (preferably a #1 AND a #2), and naked, but before I have coffee and shower. I consider this my "basal weight" for the day and therefore the best weight to compare to determine weight changes week over week.

intake of calories in each <u>meal</u> come from fat and the remainder from protein and carbs.

2. **Grams: Eat at least as many grams of fat as you do of protein in any <u>meal</u>.**

3. **Carbs: Keep your intake of carbs to 25 - 30 grams total per <u>day</u> (25 isn't a minimum – less is even better.)**

Number one is what keeps your body solidly in ketosis as carbs and protein become a much smaller component in your food intake.

If you're eating 60% of your calories as fat, then you are eating 40% of the remainder as either protein or carbohydrates. We consider this 60/40 ratio, the Golden Ratio. It is the mark we recommend you shoot for. You'll find it isn't that difficult once you overcome your old ideas about fat. In fact, we've sometimes found it hard to hold it to 60/40 and have eaten 70/30 or even 80/20. Is that bad? Not necessarily. More on this in a minute.

Number two is a guideline that will help you to eat enough protein to maintain healthy essential protein nutrition but insure eating enough fat so that you do not eat too much protein. Too much protein makes your body think you're eating too many carbs and you're suddenly back to number one again and starting over.

Number three is what actually starts to tick down the insulin levels so you can get in ketosis. And it is probably the most squirrelly of the bunch to nail down. A person's tolerance for carbs is highly individual. Unlike, say protein, there is no magic number you can say that everyone needs to stay beneath.

As we say, this doesn't happen overnight. It takes on average two weeks.

Do men lose more weight
on HFLC than women?
Umm. Yes, at least initially
but not because of the
HFLC specifics. Culturally
men spend far less time in
their life on diets than
women.

AND...

The fact is that, over your
life so far, the more times
you've dieted, quit, and
regained the weight you
lost, the more resistant
you become to losing
weight on the next diet.
So, yes, initially, men in
general lose more weight
on an HFLC diet than
women.

BUT....

No, as long as one stays on
it as a lifestyle. Everyone
will eventually settle at
what their body considers
(more or less) your ideal
weight.

For some people it can happen as quickly as a week, for others longer than two weeks.

[Reality Check: Look, we know the science says that you can actually kick up the ketones much quicker than two weeks, in fact, it happens often within 24 hours as fasting shows. (See the Special Section coming up.) But the reality is that the switch over is also dependent on the insulin levels being reduced to minimum. That, unfortunately does not happen as quickly. So we put in the "two week" caveat to keep you from getting discouraged. We know as soon as we say that, you're thinking you're part of the one week or less crowd. Maybe. But maybe not. But more to the point, if you're thinking in terms of weeks, you're thinking wrong. This is a lifestyle (i.e. for the rest of your life) decision. One week, two weeks, three weeks, whatever. You're in it for the long haul. Stop thinking like a drag racer.]

Remember, above a certain number of carbs, your body adjusts by producing more insulin to deal with them. Below that number, the pathway stays solidly dominated by ketosis. So, even if you are eating a high proportion of your daily calories as fat, and keeping your fat/protein ratio in the sweet spot, if you are eating too many carbs, the first two are really all for naught.

So can we give you a hint as to what the number for "too many grams of carbs" is? Yes, but it is just a hint. We have a general idea but each person is different.

Many sources for HFLC suggest that 50 grams of carbs per day is the maximum the majority of people can tolerate before insulin levels react and you lose the ketotic advantage.

I was fortunate to have dinner with Dr.

HFLC - a diet lifestyle where you quit worrying about weight

One of the things you will quickly realize is how much better you feel with the HFLC lifestyle. You will find yourself more alert with more energy as well as beginning to lose weight. And there are significant health benefits as well. The data seems to indicate that our bodies respond very well to higher fat intake and that our systems, including our immune systems, get more revved up.

Our experience is that most people who do HFLC, do it initially to lose weight, but they stay with it because of the general health benefits.

Eric Westman (HFLC author and researcher) one evening and I put that question to him. What is the max number of grams of carbohydrates the average person can consume and still remain in ketosis? His answer was the orthodox "50", but he spent some time emphasizing the high variability of that number.

The idea, it seems, is that if you have 50 people in a room, no two of which are the same height, you can get an average height, say 5' 10", but no one is necessarily going to be that height and there is going to be a large variability between the shortest and the tallest.

But if you have another group of 50, 25 of which are right around 5' 10" tall, you are going to have perhaps the same average, but far less variability than the first group.

Dr. Westman's suggestion was that the first case is descriptive of carb tolerance. There's an average, but that is misleading because it varies widely among individuals. He has known people who could stay in ketosis and consume 100 grams of carbohydrates per day. I personally am very carb intolerant and if I eat much above 15 grams or so, I'm in trouble.

Soooooo…

What we are going to suggest is to start with the lowest number of grams of carbs you think you can tolerate. Try less than 25. Shoot for that for the first couple of weeks. You can adjust upward from there if you want after that with 50 as the tipping point for most people. We think that most people who do HFLC tend to want to stay away from that tipping point, and wisely so. However, it is a good number to know.

Getting to ketosis faster.

Are there things you can do to get into

Do calories matter?
Yes and no.

Yes, because as you progress in the HFLC lifestyle, you want to keep tabs on the ratio of fat to protein and this is most easily done when both are calculated in terms of calories.

But, no, not in the traditional sense where you are concerned about the total number of calories you are eating and are trying to keep it to some minimum or target number (or less).
We're not saying that calories don't matter concerning weight loss. We are saying that with a high fat diet, if you do not eat beyond what it takes to satiate your appetite (which you will find easier and easier to do) you won't be eating enough calories to be concerned about.
It isn't calories that satisfy you. It is to some extent protein and to a much larger extent fat.

ketosis faster? Yes, but you're probably asking that because you want to start losing weight faster. Don't worry about that. As long as you follow those three rules, you're going to lose weight. It is inevitable.

You're going to lose water weight the first week. That's going to be good for several pounds of your body weight depending on your starting weight.

The second week you're going to lose weight just because you are going to be eating smaller portions less often. That's one of the wonderful side effects of eating more fat in your diet: it is very filling, you tend to eat less, and you tend to take longer to get hungry again. Often, by the second week, many HFLC'ers are skipping a meal, not by discipline or design, but simply because they either forget to eat them or decide they don't need them. Hunger is rarely an issue.

By the third week, your weight loss will be due to a more or less solid ketotic process. Your "Ketone Kid" will be kicking butt and you'll continue to see weight loss.

So don't worry about how long it is going to take to get into ketosis. You're going to be losing weight right along.

If you are a die hard do it yourselfer, here is what you can do to help the process along.

1. Cut out all alcohol for two weeks. Even spritzers. Any day you drink is a day you aren't going to lose weight or help your transition to ketosis. (More on this in the next chapter.)

2. Don't even think about carb cheating with "just a nibble." It isn't that the carbs will hurt you weight-wise. It is that it will slow down your transition. Your pancreas will translate the sweet as a message that carbs are "incoming" and start

A word about artificial
sweeteners
We make no endorsement
of one artificial sweetener
over another in terms of its
impact on ketosis. We're
professionals and we are
confused by a lot of the
conflicting studies on
various sweeteners we've
seen. Our hearts go out to
you if you are worried
about such things.
The best advice we can
offer is simply eat/drink as
little of it as possible, but
don't beat yourself up if
you eat/drink more than
you think you ought to.
Health-wise, our opinion is
that there are hundreds of
risks you take every day
that are more potentially
harmful than the type of
sweetener you are using in
moderation. And in our
opinion, the health
benefits of losing weight
far outweigh the risks of
judiciously using various
artificial sweeteners.
Nevertheless, let your
conscience be your guide.

revving up insulin levels. The thing about insulin as we told you earlier, is it goes up fast and comes down real slow.

3. Provided you can get enough protein to meet your daily minimum level, you can increase the ratio of fat to protein. For short spurts, you could eat a 70/30 to 80/20 fat to protein percentage ratio.

4. Stay away from artificially sweetened things for the two weeks.

We apologize in advance that we have no data on that last one as of yet, but our personal experience between the two of us is that when we eat things that are sweet, regardless of whether or not they are "low impact carbs" like sugar alcohols or sucralose (Splenda®), we get cravings for more sweet things. No one needs that during the "burn in" period of switching over from carbs to fat...really at any time. However, once you get fully on the Ketone Wagon, you'll find it much, much easier to resist that craving.

We suspect that this is indicative of our pancreas saying, "Hey, sugary things incoming" and ramping up insulin which in turn sparks our body's craving for more sweets. It's a vicious cycle that's good to avoid during that first two weeks.

Carbs, it turns out (to us at least), are habit forming and create addiction like cravings. There is a withdrawal from carbs during the first two weeks in our experience, but really that can happen anytime in the HFLC lifestyle if sweet carbs sneak in. The pancreas is constantly looking for "sugar signals" even if you've been in the HFLC lifestyle for years.

It seems like carb craving can rear it's ugly head randomly, at any time. Although, usually after some reflection, we realize it is 6-12 hours after consuming too many

Carb Craving
Carb craving revolves mostly around sweet things...sugar carbs...although we know people, ourselves included, who can find themselves craving non-sweet carbs, like hot bread or a baked potato. We suspect there is a chemical link between sweet taste and sweet cravings. However, we suspect there is no such link for starchy foods. Rather we suspect the connection is more Pavlovian than insulin. We associate feelings of warmth and comfort with those types of foods, and so we crave them when we "crave" those feelings. This probably isn't 100% infallible, but we suspect with a little introspection, most folks would find a link.

sweet tasting things. We may wonder why we have that irresistible desire for a Krispy Kreme® donut until we remember we had a couple of bottles of diet soda and a sugar free pudding last night.

Am I in ketosis? - Ketone Test Strips

OK. So back to starting up. The following question often comes up: How will you know if it's working and you're in ketosis?

The simple answer is that if you continue to lose weight and you are putting the right things in your mouth, it's automatic. You don't need to wonder.

But experience tells us that isn't enough for most people, so consider a quick trip to the drug store. Go to the prescription counter and ask for Ketone Test Strips. There are a number of companies that make them under various brand names, and the druggist or assistant will know what you're looking for. I'm not sure why they keep them behind the counter, but you don't have to sign anything or explain anything to get them.

They are impregnated with a reagent that reacts to ketones in the urine. Simply hold the end of one of them in your urine stream for a moment (not too long or the reagent can wash off giving a false negative). The bottle will have a chart to compare against the color of the reagent to determine the level of ketones.

Supposedly, the more "purple-ish" the tab turns, the more ketones there are in your urine. But in reality, any change in color means you've been successful in getting into ketosis.

Oh, but you say, it isn't really purple. It's more of a mauve.

Yeah, we get it. You want purple. Well, you're just going to have to adjust your expectations. Some people, a rare few, pee purple. Most of us pee something closer between mauve and lavender.

And that's OK. Here's why:

Urine measurement of ketones is the least accurate and most variable of all methods, but it beats sticking those needles in your finger to get blood levels, trust me. The finger prick method is much more accurate, but it is also much more complicated and much more uncomfortable and much more expensive.

And besides, all you really care is that you are in ketosis, not necessarily how far in. That's all that is really important.

The common and logical (and wrong) thought is that the more purple, the more ketotic you are, and the faster you're going to lose weight.

On some level we suppose that's true, but the reality is that ketone strips are very susceptible to what scientists call "confounds", unrelated things that can screw up results.

The color of the reagent can be influenced by the time of the day, how long ago you ate, what you ate, how much water you've drunk, how long it's been since you last went to the bathroom, how old the strip is, how long the bottle of strips has had the seal cracked, and so on.

But while they are notoriously inaccurate for measuring exact ketone levels, they are reasonably accurate from a "yes/no" perspective. You are either in ketosis or not. If there is a color change in the purple direction, you're in, regardless of how slight the change seems.

Keeping Track of Fat, Protein, and Carbs

It's already dawned on some of you that you're going to have to actually, physically,

What's the real value of ketone strips in the long run?
Once you've found out you're in ketosis, do you need ketone strips anymore?
Not really...with one exception. Many people want to "up" their carb intake from some minimum. We're not sure why people want more carbs given what we've said about carb cravings, but they do...maybe to find the "tipping point". Whatever.
Ketone strips can be helpful as an indicator of how many grams of carbs you can tolerate and still stay in ketosis. As you up your daily carb intake, check consistently with ketone strips. At some point the reagent is not going to respond. Subtract about 5 grams of your daily carb intake and that's your number.
Lifestyle-wise, you're going to want to stay well below that number. But on occasion (e.g. Thanksgiving), that's a good number to know.

religiously keep track of what goes in your mouth. Yup.

We did say you wouldn't have to count calories if you went HFLC, that's true. And that wasn't a come on. But what we meant was that you wouldn't have to maintain a calorie limit. You are going to have to count stuff.

You're going to have to count calories so that you can make sure the ratio of fat to protein and carbs is in balance. That ratio is a ratio of calories (units of energy) rather than weight (e.g. grams). You'll count grams, but you'll convert them to calories to determine the right proportions.

Second, you're going to have to count grams, mostly of carbohydrates.

Thirdly, you're going to want to write stuff down because you'll need to keep track over a day of the whole shebang. We are focused on meals, but often we snack, nosh, and pick a lot. That's all got to be factored in, too.

You can go analog and low tech by carrying around a physical paper diary. You'll need to also carry a food/nutrient encyclopedic resource of some kind, too, so you know exactly what you're eating.

There's nothing wrong with this early 20th century method other than for men it is inconveniently bulky with no purse or bag. You'll end up with stickies or slips of paper which will have to be entered in a diary somewhere before the end of the day. For us, that's been a show stopper for the diary method.

The encyclopedic resource is a good idea though, no matter what recording method you use. Make sure it is one that deals with common foods in normal portion sizes and breaks the components down into calories, carbs, fat, and protein. One of the best we've ever used is

Am I Entering a Life of Carb Counting?

Let's be frank here. "I lost weight by not paying attention to my food intake." said no one, ever. A key part of your lifestyle change is going to have to be that you make conscious decisions about what you do and do not put in your mouth. Otherwise, no change in diet is ever going to produce the results you want.

So, yes, you are entering a life of paying attention to food. But, no, you are not going to have to count carbs forever. But, yes, you do have to, from time to time, count carbs between now and forever. Go back and read the chapter on hidden carbs. Lack of some level of diligence happens to everyone over time, and the only cure is to start paying attention again.

published annually, can be purchased online or in most bookstores, and has the added advantage of including information on most supermarket brands and major restaurant chain servings. The Calorie King: Calorie, Fat, & Carbohydrate Counter by Allan Borushek. You'll definitely want to add this to your library.

The real value of having a book like this even if you go digital is that it allows you to browse through it to educate yourself on what is and is not consistent with a HFLC lifestyle. And Borushek's inclusion of the analysis of both brand name grocery items and national chain restaurant dishes is incredibly helpful in locating what you should and shouldn't eat.

Now as to your food journal/diary...yes, you can go analog. But if you have a smart phone or use a computer we highly recommend a free app called Lose It! It is available in multiple formats to fit most operating systems and, like The Calorie King, it has an encyclopedic reservoir of data on a huge variety of foods, home made, store bought, and restaurant brands. You simply find the food you just ate, choose the right portion size, and Lose It! does the rest. It automatically keeps track of protein, fat, and carbs.

In addition, you can enter any food you don't find in their nearly exhaustive index, "recipes" for stuff you make yourself (like some of the ones at the end of this book), and if you eat the same meal day after day, you can copy meals from one day to the next.

Finally, failing all of that, if what you're eating comes out of a package with a bar code, Lose It! allows you to scan the barcode with your phone's camera, and it will look up the nutritional information in its data base.

Developing Discipline
Probably the major reason
lifestyle changes fail is a
lack of discipline. Eating is
regular. Therefore, like it
or not, eating is a habit. Or
more to the point, what
you eat is a habit.

And to this the fact that
sweet foods definitely
have an addictive quality
(the more you eat, the
more you want), and you
must admit what you've
been eating up to this
point is a self reinforcing
habit of obese proportions.

THEREFORE: the greater
the habit, the more
discipline and energy it is
going to take to break it
and replace it with
another, better habit.

That's the bad news. The
good news is that at some
point (as we've found out
personally) eating healthy
becomes a habit, too, and
doesn't require the
ongoing effort to stay the
course. Take heart. It gets
easier.

It also has the ability for you to enter your weight to track it over time. And we've only scratched the surface as to features.

That's it! You're on your way. Armed with knowledge, apps, books, and your own commitment, get ready for change for the good.

What could possibly go wrong, right?

Well, the title of this book is The Straight Skinny and we've been trying to tell you the truth up to this point. No sense in stopping now.

A lot can go wrong, and for most of us, it usually does at some point. So the next section will attempt to answer the question of why bad things happen to good people living an HFLC lifestyle.

Special Section

GETTING THE SHAKES!

two aids to getting and staying in the HFLC lifestyle

Everything in Chapter 6 that you've read is correct. And if you follow the 3 keys to the HLFC lifestyle, that's really all you need. We promised we'd simplify it for you, and we did.

However...

As you probably thought, there are some things that we've discovered over the years to jump start the lifestyle. Also, in Chapter 7 we're going to share some secrets around how to recover from the inevitable plateaus and slumps.

But if you're just starting out, you're not at a plateau or in a slump. You're just excited about the potential and ready to "rock and roll."

So here are two things we think can make your transition from your old lifestyle to your new one easier.

Getting the Shakes!

Learning how to cook in the HFLC manner will come naturally, but it does take time to learn and experiment with. The first few days eating cheese omelets cooked in real butter with a side of bacon is going to be liberating, no doubt.

The temptation will be there to have ribeye (one of the fattiest cuts of meat) every night with mashed cauliflower slathered in butter and a small tossed salad dripping with olive oil.

Yup. All good.

But while you're learning all this, there is a short cut you can take that will both help jump start your ketotic state AND make your hectic life a tad easier to manage: an HLFC Shake.

It's not a brand name, but just something we call what others call protein shakes. Protein shakes emphasize the protein content for high performance athletes and tend to cater to a low fat lifestyle. We've taken the idea and modified it a bit to adjust the protein to fat ratio to levels we think are better for the HLFC lifestyle by boosting the fat content to actually exceed that "magic" ratio.

Why? Well, the idea is that you can replace a meal with a shake that is quick and easy to make, delicious, and as satisfying as the meal it replaces.

And it has the added benefit that as you substitute shakes for a meal, fewer carbs "sneak in" so your weight loss goals become more reachable faster.

There's a recipe for the shake in Chapter 9, but we'll cover the basics here.

The first step is finding a protein shake powder that is right for you. We like the powder/instant idea because it is easy to use, easy to store, and easy to take with you when you travel.

There are a ton of protein shakes on the market. We don't care which brand you decide on, but our preference is that you select one that is made with whey protein isolate rather than soy protein isolate.

Whey, as the name suggests, comes from milk and is an animal protein. The soy is a protein derived from soy beans and so is a vegetable protein. Our preference is for animal proteins, but the call is yours.

Obviously you'll also want to select one with low or no carbs. That should reduce a bunch of choices down to a manageable number.

Our favorites are Isopure and Pure Protein. We are not endorsing these brands or recommending them. These are just the two we use as we have found them to be consistently good tasting, easy to use, and available in a ton of flavor choices (including unflavored).

You can get them in some health food stores, occasionally in the health food section of some larger drug store chains, but more consistently online. We order the 3lb. plastic jug, but you can get them in a variety of sizes.

The directions on the jug assumes you are an athlete looking for a low fat protein supplement. So the manufacturer recommends mixing the powder with water or juices.

As a meal replacement for HFLC, that would violate the three keys...and set you up for the main way people stumble on the HFLC lifestyle: failure to consume enough fat.

What we recommend is using only part of the water the directions call for and using good old heavy cream (your new friend) for the rest...and maybe add even a bit more for taste.

If you've picked an ice cream related flavor (e.g. chocolate, coffee, etc.) the result is going to have the consistency of and taste just like an old fashioned milk shake.

Our recipe is simple. Take a scoop of the protein powder (the scoop comes with it), 5 fluid ounces of cold water, and 3 fluid ounces of heavy cream. Mix until creamy/frothy with an immersion blender and drink.

With this mixture, the shake generates a meal replacement that is 86% fat and almost 14% protein. And because you are using heavy cream, the fat is mostly what are called a "medium chain triglyceride" which is the easiest type of fat for your body to instantly recognize and use for energy without having to invest a lot of time and resources into making it something more useable.

In short, it is a fat jump start to your lifestyle, made up of readily usable fuel for your body, which will create a sense of long lasting satisfaction.

It isn't a lot in the glass. In fact, you'll look at it and doubt it will do much to stave of cravings, let alone fill you up after drinking it. But once you down it, you will be surprised at how satisfied you feel. Hours later, you will realize how "unhungry" you are compared to how you felt on your previous lifestyle diet.

We've learned to make these shakes a regular part of our day. In fact, Dr. Simonds coaches his clients that if you want to easily maintain your weight losses, drink one shake a day. If you want to increase your weight losses, drink two shakes a day.

On occasion when we both have wanted to break the back of some bad carb habits that had crept back in to our lifestyle, we gone for a long as a week to 10 days eating nothing but 3 shakes a day.

The table that follows shows the results on one 10 day trial. From a weight perspective we each lost about 6-7% of our starting weight (a little over a pound a day for each of us). That's remarkable for a 10 day period. However, even more remarkable, from a "cravings" perspective, our carb cravings were essentially eliminated within the first 48 hours. And probably most remarkable, neither of us felt like we were hungry or really missed other types of food for the period. Our bodies were satiated and our mental and emotional status was excellent.

Weigh in morning of	Lbs Lost				% Lost			
	Wickham		Skip		Wickham		Skip	
	Daily	Cumulative	Daily	Cumulative	Daily	Cumulative	Daily	Cumulative
Day 1								
Day 2	2.2	2.2	1.6	1.6	0.98%	0.98%	0.84%	0.84%
Day 3	4.4	6.6	2.6	4.2	1.96%	2.94%	1.37%	2.21%
Day 4	0.8	7.4	1.4	5.6	0.36%	3.30%	0.74%	2.95%
Day 5	2.0	9.4	1.6	7.2	0.89%	4.19%	0.84%	3.79%
Day 6	0.8	10.2	0.6	7.8	0.36%	4.55%	0.32%	4.11%
Day 7	0.2	10.4	0.8	8.6	0.09%	4.64%	0.42%	4.53%
Day 8	0.8	11.2	1.8	10.4	0.36%	5.00%	0.95%	5.47%
Day 9	0.8	12.0	0.0	10.4	0.36%	5.35%	0.00%	5.47%
Day 10 - Final	2.8	14.8	-0.4	10.0	1.25%	6.60%	-0.21%	5.26%
Average Daily	1.6		1.1		0.7%		0.6%	

We've done these regimens on many occasions and the results are always largely the same. We lost weight, we conquered carb cravings, we were not hungry, and we felt great.

Are we recommending a 7 or 10 day shake trial for you? Nope. We are not recommending it. We offer it only as an "in vivo" illustration of the power of incorporating HFLC shakes into your new lifestyle.

What we are recommending is that you consider incorporating at least one shake a day into your daily regimen. You'll be glad you did.

Slow Down Fast!

It is no secret that obesity is one of the great health concerns of our times. At the time of writing, the most recent statistics indicate that more than 70% of adults in the US are overweight or obese. (https://www.niddk.nih.gov/health-information/health-statistics/overweight-obesity)

One of the areas we have been looking at is the growing awareness of weight gain and obesity as a disease rather than a benign state. We've known for years that weight gain beyond a certain point is not healthy. And the science around this seems to be indicating that like any disease, being obese or overweight over time produces relatively intractable changes to your system that resist attempts to lose weight and keep it off. In short, the excess weight changes your body in ways that promote and accept weight gain as the new norm.

It seems once obesity has reached a certain point, that your body not only accepts it as "normal" but it tends to fight to maintain it in the face of weight loss. As you lose weight the body fights it and when you reach a stasis, like a goal or determine you don't want to diet anymore, your body begins an almost inevitable process of using and allocating resources to reverse the weight loss...plus adding in a little more.

It is this setting of the body's definition of what is a "normal" condition that is so disease like. Diseases tend to overwhelm a healthy body and use the body's resources to protect and promote itself at the expense of the body. This is definitely what obesity does.

One of the nice things about a lifestyle change is that it gives you the life long strategy to put up an ongoing resistance to this regression, and by continued good choices, maintain your new body weight. But even for those of us who for years have been able to maintain weight loss, we are aware that the fight to stay at or near goal is subtle but never ending. Our body isn't embracing our reduced weight as "healthy" in a sense, and is constantly looking for a way to add pounds back on.

So the question is: can the body's metabolic "perspective" be "reset". Can we reset the weight counter to our new weight so that our bodies quit trying to sabotage us?

We think so. And we think the key is fasting - either caloric restrictions on a periodic basis or complete fasting for periods between 6 and 24 hours.

The emerging science is beginning to support this idea. For example, researchers at the University of Florida have found that intermittent fasting can help "flip' the switch between fat storage and fat consumption by the body.

To quote from the outcomes of that study:

"Emerging findings suggest that the metabolic switch from glucose to fatty acid-derived ketones represents an evolutionarily conserved trigger

point that shifts metabolism from lipid/cholesterol synthesis and fat storage to mobilization of fat through fatty acid oxidation and fatty acid-derived ketones, which serve to preserve muscle mass and function. Thus, IF [Intermittent Fasting] regimens that induce the metabolic switch have the potential to improve body composition in overweight individuals. Moreover, IF regimens also induce the coordinated activation of signaling pathways that optimize physiological function, enhance performance, and slow aging and disease processes."
(https://onlinelibrary.wiley.com/doi/10.1002/oby.22065)

It is that last phrase that is of particular interest here: fasting induces "the coordinated activation of signaling pathways that optimize physiological function…." To us, that sounds a lot like reseting the system.

The primary researcher in this study, Stephen D. Anton, PhD, made the following statement when interviewed about this study.

"An important takeaway is that we all have the ability to switch our metabolism from glucose to ketone utilization. And that switch has the potential to have profound health benefits for us, in addition to the positive changes in body composition."
(https://www.medicalnewstoday.com/articles/321690.php)

We agree.

The idea of fasting has been around from time immemorial. Read ancient religious texts and you'll find fasting was commanded and considered a regular part of the lifestyle expected of the people. Certain days of the year were set aside for fasting. When certain calamities were threatening, fasts were called. Fasting was considered on a par with praying.

In our 21st Century lifestyle, I dare say the vast majority of Americans have never purposely fasted. And even religious folks tend to look a fasting as a sort of activity of "last resort."

But what if fasting was actually good for you? What if going completely without food or only eating meals with a significant caloric restriction on a regular basis for anywhere from 6 hours to a day...a 24 hour period...actually did something good?

Dr. Simonds has talked in the past that fasting may actually be the key to resetting your metabolic default weight.

We'll need a bit more science before we incorporate fasting wholesale into the HFLC lifestyle. But it is close.

Realize we're not talking about long term, multi-day, and total abstinence giving up of food. What we are talking about is:

- regular
- relatively frequent
- short duration fasts

- of 6 to 24 hours
- with either total abstinence of food or a highly restricted caloric intake.

Our feeling is that the effectiveness of the fast is going to be its regularity (we think once a week is good, but 2 or 3 times is even better if you can do it regularly), its length (we favor longer over shorter), and the content.

The science seems to indicate that the more often you fast (alternate day fasting seems to be the max) and the closer to abstinence you can get will have the greater impact as opposed to a single, weekly 6 hour fast with caloric restrictions. There appears to be a spectrum of benefit between those two.

It is clear, however, that any fasting is better than none. So, if the best you can do is a 6 hour caloric restriction every now and again, you go!

As always, you should check with your physician about whether fasting presents any concerns for you. Don't make a decision to fast based on a book. Get input from your physician.

Also, it may be helpful to print out the study we cited for your physician to review. It is likely that he or she is already aware of it, but it wouldn't hurt to have a copy with you.

Clearly it appears there is something to this fasting thing. And as we have realized ourselves, if nothing else, it is definitely a way to demonstrate to ourselves that we have control over our appetites rather than our appetites having control over us. But now there appears to be major health benefits as well.

7

ALCOHOL AND HIDDEN CARBS
and other speed bumps on the road to success

Part of the goal of this book is to cut through the politically correct fluff that many diet books have to include to be acceptable to publishers and readers. So we've spent a fair amount of time talking about your biological processes and metabolic pathways and other such scientific stuff to help you feel comfortable with one really simple idea: fat is your friend.

Unfortunately, in building that case, we recognize that it can sound like a HFLC diet can be a "foolproof" method for losing weight and maintaining that weight loss over time in a healthy manner.

Well, as we all know, they are always inventing better fools, so there is nothing that is truly "fool proof". And the authors themselves are cases in point. We've figured out, over the years, how to sabotage this lifestyle fairly well.

So the purpose of this chapter is to talk about some of the road blocks and speed bumps that we and others have run into, and to help you understand why. We believe if you understand why certain things create issues, it will be easier for you to avoid them.

Question #1
Can I drink if I'm doing HFLC?

Sure, assuming you would be drinking if you weren't doing the HFLC lifestyle. Obviously if you have problems with alcohol, the HFLC lifestyle isn't going to solve those problems. But in general, yes, you can have adult beverages.

There was a diet popular back in the fifties called "The Drinking Man's Diet". In many ways it was similar to the HFLC diet and has been making a bit of a come back of late.

While we agree that the diet part of it is sound, we have a bit of a problem with the alcohol part. Oh, the diet worked back in the day, but we are less sure of its efficacy today. And the reason for that has nothing to do with the diet itself, but much more to do with the time in which it was put forth.

Back when it was originally published, the most frequently occurring job in the United States was industrial/manufacturing. And as you'll see in this chapter, physical activity can have an impact on the speed with which your body processes alcohol.

We don't think in today's "information age" the diet has the same impact.

But...

And you knew that was coming. Consuming alcohol does impact the effects of the HFLC diet, in fact any diet, on you. Here's the rough rule of thumb and then we'll give you all the caveats.

Any day you drink is a day you are not going to lose weight.

Now you may or may not gain weight on that day, but almost for sure, you aren't going to lose weight. So if losing weight is the goal, probably you would want to reduce the number of days you drink until you lose the weight you want to lose.

OK, here come the caveats:

1. There is a tremendous amount of personal variability in the way each person responds to alcohol. To our knowledge there are no really solid scientific studies on this topic (alcohol and HFLC) but in Dr. Simonds' practice, the standard seems to be that there is no standard. Some people tend to tolerate alcohol better than others. But in general, everyone experiences a pause in weight loss with alcohol.

2. We are assuming you would be drinking beverages that have little or no carb content. If what you're drinking is sugary after dinner liquors, mixed drinks using fruit juice and/or sugar syrups, or alcohol flavored with various things that have carbs, all bets are off. But then the problem is less the alcohol and more the carbs you're consuming.

3. Drinking any alcohol to excess does two very dangerous things besides the obvious dangers that come with that. First, alcohol stimulates your hunger centers. That's not necessarily a problem, but when combined with the second thing, alcohol reduces your inhibitions, the two form a "1-2 punch" that is often a killer in any diet,

We are not espousing drinking. In fact, if pressed, we think drinking and long term health are often at odds.

However, we are realists and understand that we live in a society where drinking alcohol is often a social expectation.

So our goal here is to help you make good choices about alcohol through understanding how your body deals with it.

And we also want to manage your expectations around weight loss.

So, bottom line, if you can get away with not drinking alcohol when you are in the weight loss period of your lifestyle change, don't drink.

and especially a low carb diet. Fact: if you drink and especially if you drink a lot, you are more likely to make poor food choices that are going to put your diet and lifestyle in jeopardy.

So what is really going on in your body with this alcohol thing? Please realize that what we are about to share with you is essentially the same regardless of how you get your alcohol, whether through mixed drinks, wine, beer, or other alcoholic beverages.

We need to emphasize again that there is very little solid scientific evidence around this topic, but what follows can best be included under the caveat: "most experts agree...."

Your body prefers alcohol over all other macronutrients. So when you drink alcohol, your body shoves aside the carbs, fat, and protein you are eating in favor of processing the alcohol. That's part of the reason we say you aren't going to lose weight any day you drink.

Alcohol is a readily digestible energy source, but that isn't the only reason your body prefers it. The other reason is more defensive. Your body considers alcohol a toxin.

[tox·in ′täksən/ noun - a poison or venom of plant or animal origin, causing disease when present at low concentration in the body.]

So when we say your body "prefers" it, we're not saying it actually wants it. Instead it is more like your body gives it priority because it is a toxin and your body needs to break it down into a non-toxic form.

And that non-toxic form is acetate, which is a form which your body treats like glucose.

51

There are rules to
drinking?
Well, yes, if your goal in
changing your lifestyle is to
attain a healthy body
weight and maintain it.

In general, alcohol does
not aid or support that
goal. So before you start
drinking, you'd better have
internalized a few
important rules. You've
likely heard these before,
but they bear repeating.

1. Drink the minimum,
   not the maximum you
   can.
2. Drink slowly. Your
   body prefers its toxins
   in small, slow doses so
   it can dispose of them.
   A drink an hour is a
   good rule of thumb.
   Ask for your drink on
   the rocks (hard
   alcohol) or in a glass
   (beer). The rocks slow
   you down. The glass
   let's you see what
   you're drinking.
3. Ask for a glass of
   water with your drink,
   even if it is beer or
   wine. A lot of drinking
   is just habit (picking up
   whatever is in front of
   you from time to time)
   and having water as
   an option helps.

Fortunately, acetate does not appear to cause an insulin reaction, so if your predominant metabolic pathway is ketosis, you aren't going to "flip" out of it. It is our experience that drinking puts the state of ketosis into a "pause mode" until the acetate has been metabolized. Again a caveat is needed here. We say acetate "does not appear to cause an insulin reaction" with the accent on "appears". No one really knows if this is strictly speaking true. There isn't enough science known to really understand the interaction. We base this statement on our own general observations with ourselves and our patients.

Regardless, as we said, your body is going to postpone the digestion of fats (and carbs and protein, too) in favor of dealing with the toxin of alcohol. Hence, no weight loss is the likely outcome for that day.

As we said, the impact of alcohol is highly variable and it is difficult to predict any one person's responses. While we know that alcohol causes everyone's metabolism to shift toward breaking down the alcohol, how long that process takes, and how quickly you get back to your regular metabolism is really only determined by trial and error on a case by case basis.

We do know that activity levels have an impact on that timetable. Generally people who have a more active lifestyle tend to metabolize alcohol more quickly. Now we are NOT saying that if you drink, you can speed up the absorption process by walking vigorously for an hour, for example. That will likely have zero impact on your absorption rate.

However, if you are engaged in an active lifestyle, like a manual laborer or some other demanding occupation, you likely do have higher energy demands which would, in fact, speed up the alcohol breakdown.

In general though, most research (and there isn't a lot) seems to suggest that it takes about an hour to an hour and a half to deal with one drink. This is a gross oversimplification, but is a rule of thumb we feel somewhat confident in.

So then you'll ask, if you drink and wait an hour or so before eating a meal; would that avoid the "non-weight loss" day thing?

Theoretically (and we are not advocating this), yes. BUT remember that "1-2 punch": when you drink you simultaneously stimulate hunger pangs and reduce your ability to make good food choices.

So aside from the fact you'd have to start that martini at 3:30pm in the afternoon to avoid the "hit" on your 6pm dinner, you probably aren't going to wait that long for dinner in the first place. Or overeat if you do.

Bottom line: you can drink, but adjust your expectations that your low carb diet is going to be bullet proof.

Question #2
Why am I no longer losing weight? I'm doing HFLC!

This is something that happens a lot to folks who are using the HFLC lifestyle as a means to lose weight. Initially weight begins to drop off and life is good. Then somewhere along the line, the weight loss slows down and occasionally stops. What's up with that?

Well, there are a few possible reasons. Let's take them in order of least likely to most likely.

Everyone, regardless of the strategy they use for losing weight, experiences a period of time (more likely periods, plural) where weight loss stops and even occasionally reverses. There are basically two causes for this. One is good, and you can't do much about it. The other is bad, but you can do something about it.

The good pause is when your body is "shifting gears". It has been shedding fat, learning a new lifestyle, becoming acclimated to different food choices. At some point, it requires time to move from one "level" to another. Not much you can do about this but wait it out.

The other is when you start sabotaging yourself. That's what this section is about. You'll see there are solutions.

Which is you? We recommend you assume it is the bad type, eliminate the causes, and whatever is left has to be good.

1, *Equilibrium*

Maybe you've reached a weight where your body has decided it is happy and has acclimated to your new lifestyle. Further weight loss is only going to be possible with significant changes in your exercise regimen, and possibly your food intake.

This does happen to all of us who are "lifers" with the HFLC lifestyle. So why have we made it the least likely answer to this question? Simply because this weight is so close to what you normally consider ideal, that you typically aren't asking the question above as your weight loss slows to a stop. So if you're asking that question, that suggests you are nowhere near goal or ideal weight.

But, for the sake of education, let's say you've been in the HFLC lifestyle for a while, and your body is in good shape, your food intake seems to be on an even keel with no significant ups or downs, and your weight yields a body mass index in the "normal" range (i.e. under 25). In this state, your body has become efficient in using the energy you are consuming for your energy needs of daily life. So if you want to lose more weight, you are going to need to adopt a more energetic lifestyle. And we aren't talking about just doing an extra yoga class a week. To permanently up your body's need for energy, you are going to need a daily change.

We're not saying that extra yoga class isn't going to be good for you. To the contrary, it will be good. But anything short of a daily energy demand isn't going to shift your body back into a metabolic rate that will consume more energy than what you are eating.

Now that either isn't possible for some folks, or for whatever reason, that answer is less than ideal. If I can't increase my daily

Recently there has been a spate of news reports about the results of laboratory tests on rats where they are fed "starvation" diets. The results indicate that these rats, subsisting on very low calorie diets (VERY low calorie diets), live longer than rats that eat a regular diet of whatever lab rats eat.

The conclusion we are tempted to jump to is that very low calorie diets may actually make us live longer. And wouldn't that be a good thing?

The problem with this type of thinking is that lab rats can only eat what they are given to eat. You, on the other hand, have to choose what you eat several times a day, each and every day. The psycho-social energy cost to you to do that is great. And we wonder if that doesn't more than off set any health benefits.

activities, what else is available to me? If it is equilibrium, can you just eat less instead of exercising more?

Theoretically yes, but there is a law of diminishing returns here. In equilibrium your body is satisfied with what you're eating, and presumably you are, too, since it took you a while to get to this point. So anything you do in terms of adjusting your daily food intake downward is going to change that, and our experience says that isn't likely to be a strategy you'll maintain going forward for very long. Eventually you'll find yourself eating what you're eating now, and your weight will be back to this point.

And there are also health concerns around eating too little.

Again, our experience is that folks who have been on a HFLC lifestyle for a while (months if not years) tend to eat smaller portions by choice (because high fat meals are very satisfying) and usually don't eat between meals (because they are rarely hungry between meals for the same reason). In fact, some of us have that blissful experience from time to time where we realize we forgot to eat a meal because our body wasn't sending us hunger pangs.

So if your weight "pause" is equilibrium and your body is already eating judiciously, reducing food intake may create a nutrient deficit you neither want nor need because there may be health ramifications. We don't recommend this as a worthwhile strategy for permanent additional weight loss.

2, *The "low fat" version of a HFLC lifestyle*

Educating Your Friends and Family about Carbs

OK, you get it: carbs and calories are not the same thing. But your friends and family think counting carbs is the same as counting calories. "Here, eat this. You can catch up later." Or "It's good to splurge now and again."

Basically you've got two choices. One is to eat it or pretend to eat it. We think that's a bad choice. If you eat it, you run the risk of flipping out of your fat burning mode for several days AND you encourage them to serve you the same at another time. If you pretend to eat it, you risk your host thinking you didn't like what they prepared. Neither is good.

The other choice is to just say, "No, thank you." They'll ask why in one form or another. And the answer is simply, "I'm trying to cut these foods out of my diet."

In the long run, friends and family will get the message AND respect you more for your self-discipline.

Sometimes we carry over some "old school" thinking into our "new school" HFLC lifestyle. You'll notice that we don't talk a lot about calories. There's a couple of reasons for that. One is that folks often tend to think of calories and grams of carbohydrates as interchangeable concepts.

For example, if you are not doing a HFLC lifestyle and are essentially going "old school" by counting calories, you know that if you have a daily intake goal of, say, 1500 calories, you can occasionally over eat and make up for it the next meal or the next day by eating proportionally fewer calories.

Not so with carbohydrates, because carbs are what control insulin production, so overeating carbs can possibly trigger a significant enough rise in your insulin levels that you get thrown out of that ketotic state and have long multi-day process of getting back into it. Overeating carbs can't be off set by under eating carbs the next meal or day.

So we don't talk a lot about calories because we want you to stay focused on carb intake as that is the key to burning fat.

The other reason we don't talk about calories is that when you are burning fat, your body is less sensitive to the number of calories you eat. It isn't that calories are irrelevant or unimportant. It is just that when your body is in fat burning mode, it is a whole lot more efficient in using the calories you eat, all of them, and far less likely to store them as body fat. In fact, that's the whole point of the HFLC lifestyle is to get into that fat burning mode so that your body becomes so efficient at burning fat, you regularly burn more energy than you consume.

BUT, old thinking is hard to break, and all of us (and I mean all of us, including the

Reminder: Lifestyle versus Diet

Folks, remember you are making a lifestyle change. That means this is a permanent adjustment to your way of eating. That means you are committing to this regardless of circumstances.

That means you have to be patient when you hit plateaus or even occasionally regain weight you've already lost.

Patience is probably one of the major outcomes of making a lifestyle choice. If you are impatient, that is probably a strong indication that you have not fully committed to this new lifestyle because your decision is still contingent on "results". And when those results aren't there, you are rethinking your lifestyle choices.

Stop it!

authors) have found ourselves in the situation where our weight loss has plateaued and we are wondering what we can do to help it get started again.

And because we know that fat has more than twice the calories per gram of either protein or carbs, we reason that if we eat less fat, then we'll sort of "help our body along" by giving it less fat to burn.

The thinking is that if I've been losing weight with my caloric intake being X (whatever it happens to be based on your HFLC food choices - remember you are not selecting foods based on calories, but rather on maintaining the balance of fat to protein and with carbs below your trigger point), then if I eat less than X by reducing the grams of fat I'm eating, and if my activity level stays constant, I should go back to losing weight.

This is "old school". And we've all found that while it is very logical and seems like it ought to work, it doesn't. In fact, if we are measuring our fat burning rate (through ketone strips or blood tests), we find the rate lessening. In the vernacular, if we were "peeing purple", we start peeing more mauve. (Those of you who use "pee strips" will totally get this.)

Why? Why doesn't this strategy work?

The simple answer is because by eating a lower fat version of a HFLC lifestyle you are, without intending to, increasing the proportion of protein you are eating relative to fat. And if you'll refer back to the chapter on how your body handles macronutrients, you'll remember there is a discussion there of how eating too much protein relative to fat can actually throw you out of fat burning mode even though your carbohydrate intake is still below the trigger point.

It is worth mentioning at
this juncture in your
consideration of whether
you are eating hidden
carbs or not, that there is a
reverse corollary to "fat is
your friend".

"Sweet is your enemy."

We admit we have no
science for this, but based
on our and our clients'
reports, even if the
sweetening agent used in
various foods is
guaranteed not to create
an insulin response
(artificial sweeteners and
sugar alcohols, for
example) we have found
that just the "sweetness"
of the food can create a
subtle but undeniable
"craving" for more of the
same.

What starts out as one
sugar free, low carb sweet
snack/desert the first day,
becomes two the second,
and so on.

Our view is that you need
to avoid the first "sweet".
That solves the problem.

Bam! That's why you've plateaued. You're eating the wrong balance and defeating the purpose of going high fat.

Don't be hard on yourself. We've all done it. Just go back to making sure your fat and protein intake is balanced and your carbs are below the trigger point. You'll find you'll break through that plateau soon enough. Be patient.

3. Hidden carbs

OK. Here we are at the most likely explanation for your plateau. You've been losing weight, you've been feeling good and have plenty of energy. You've been buying new clothes and enjoying the compliments of friends and family about the "new you." And you've stopped paying attention to the food you're eating.

Hey, it happens.

Through no bad intentions, you've slipped into a mindset that says "I've got this" and slowly but surely your food choices have been being made with less and less concern for avoiding carbs.

Remember when you first started on this journey and carbs were like "the enemy" and you religiously sought them out and banished them from your daily diet? Man, you were all over it. In fact, truth be told, you were a little annoying to your friends and family by your rabid unwillingness to make any food or meal choice that contained any carbs, or certainly the least number of grams possible.

But somewhere along the line, you didn't go back to a high carb lifestyle, but unwanted carbs begin to sneak in to your diet unknowingly.

Maybe it started with those "low carb" snack bars. Maybe it happened when you begin to eat out more and assumed the chicken salad was just chicken, mayo, and some seasonings (not realizing that sugar was being added). Maybe your mom or wife just started adding higher carb options into the cooking regimen, rationalizing it because they (unlike you) think carbs and calories are interchangeable, and if you ate too many carbs at this meal, you can make up for it next time by eating fewer.

There are a myriad of possibilities here, but they all add up to the same problem: slowly but surely carbs have crept back into your daily food choices and you are back up to a daily carb intake that is too close to "the tipping point". Your fat burning mode has slowed, and maybe, just maybe you are actually flipped out of it all together.

The problem is that in today's food industry, carbs are a default commodity, a given, even a necessity. Ketchup has sugar in it, for heaven's sake! "All natural" products are made with "pure cane sugar" but you wouldn't think so. Even "sugar free" doesn't mean that it is low carb because the sugar has likely been replaced with honey or agave or some other "natural" sugar.

So it is almost inevitable that carbs will sneak back in unwatched for. We know. We're pros and we've been there, too.

What's a body to do?

Unfortunately, there is no substitute for good old fashioned, vigilant, unrelenting carb counting as part of a larger effort in regularly (and by "regularly" we mean, meal by meal) tracking your nutrient intake.

Yup. Count the grams of fat, carbohydrates, and protein you eat every meal, every day, for as long as it takes to get a handle on what you are actually consuming. And honestly we think that is going to take at least two weeks, minimum. Minimum. A month is better. Ongoing

Online Nutrition Info
As you get serious about
tracking your
macronutrient
consumption, you'll need
all the help you can get.

One online resource we
use a lot is:

nutritiondata.self.com

This resource provides
nutritional information in
the same format as the
nutrition labels you find in
stores.

And you can vary the
portion size to get the right
information for the portion
you are eating.

We recommend you make
it a "favorite" for your
browser.

isn't unreasonable.

In the last chapter we recommended a smart phone solution: "LoseIt". We like it because it offers a nifty breakdown of macronutrients consumed by snack or meal item choice. And it rolls those up into meal totals, day totals, and even week totals so you can get a longer term view of your food choices.

The other nifty thing that LoseIt does is to access its own database of hundreds of thousands of generic foods broken down into their constituent macronutrients saving you in most cases from having to enter the nutritional data from the food labels yourself. In addition, it contains specific breakdowns for name brand items you often buy in grocery stores as well as menu items for most national restaurant chains. Want to know the carbs in a McDonald's Egg McMuffin? LoseIt has it.

There are other apps out there. We aren't recommending one over another. Use whatever works for you. Just choose one that enables you to track your macronutrients accurately.

And then do it.

We are very confident you will be surprised by the number of hidden carbs you are eating on a regular basis. And as your food choices adjust accordingly, your fat burning process will rev up, and you'll bust through that plateau with flying colors.

Question #3

I've eliminated that my lack of continued weight loss is due to alcohol consumption, equilibrium, "low fat" HFLC, or hidden carbs. What else could it be?

There are two possibilities here. As we said earlier, one is that your body is just taking a natural "pause" in the weight loss

Dr. Brown's Weight Loss
Prescription
*"Get up offa that thing,
And dance till you feel
better.
Get up off that thing,
Try to release the pressure.*

*Get up offa that thing,
And twist till you feel
better.
Get up offa that thing,
Try to release the pressure.*

*Get up offa that thing,
And shake till you feel
better.
Get up offa that thing,
Try to release the
pressure."*

...James Brown

We couldn't agree more
with Dr. Brown.

process and will resume a higher level of metabolism shortly. Just be patient. It isn't at all unusual to hit a plateau for even a week or more. If you are doing all the right things the right way, hang in and hang on. You'll resume weight loss soon enough. Remember, this is a lifestyle choice you are in, not a diet you are on. OK?

The other possibility is that you are just too sedentary. Yes, you'll lose weight with a HFLC lifestyle, but you may not get to your goal weight if you don't "get up offa that thing" (to quote James Brown).

Changing poor food choices can take care of some of your weight issues, but you've got to also change some poor lifestyle and activity choices, to take care of the rest.

As people who have struggled with our weight in the past and even as HFLC adherents, we've tried a number of different strategies ourselves. We wouldn't presume to recommend one over another for you, especially if you are coming from a place of morbid obesity. You may actually need to lose some weight first before changing your exercise regimen (or even introducing one). If your body mass index is north of 35, when to start exercising, what exercises to do, and how much/long to do them are all real good questions for a discussion to have with your personal physician.

But for the rest of us, if we have hit a plateau and ruled out all the previous potential causes (and I don't mean you just read them and said, "Nah, that's not me."), then its time to step up to a more active lifestyle.

When Calories Count

One of the hallmarks of a LCHF diet is the elimination of the need for conscious portion control (which is a strategy for counting calories). With an HFLC diet, as we've discussed, we can rely on our decreased appetite and hunger to limit intake to appropriate levels. We just don't want to eat more than we should.

However, there are times when our bodies develop a "mind of their own" about eating. Historically there have always been folks who lived an "aesthetic" life style (monks, prophets in the wilderness, guru's on mountain tops, etc.) and there is a reason that type of lifestyle has survived at least on mountain tops. It's because every once in a while we need to take charge of our body rather than letting our body continually take charge of us. Periodic self control can break those runaway urges to eat more than we should.

Skip's experience: When I finally got serious about weight loss thanks to Dr. Simonds (see the Preface), I also decided to get serious about "getting in shape", not just losing weight. I started going to yoga two days a week...three whenever my schedule would allow. In addition, I live on the coast and purchased a small row boat and made the commitment to row 30 minutes a day. Between those two regimens, I know that not only helped me avoid a lot of the plateaus I would have undoubtedly faced, but I also was able to shape my body into a reasonably fit looking thing. I'm no Mr. Universe, for sure. But my coordination, balance, strength, and endurance have all improved.

Dr. Simonds' experience: Even though my practice keeps me focused on weight loss and maintaining weight loss almost 24/7, I struggle with plateaus and "pause points" like everyone else. Over the years I've learned two strategies that help me break through. One is actually counting calories, the other is increasing my activity level in the right way for weight loss.

While I don't recommend counting calories as a means of ongoing weight loss and maintaining weight loss, for me there are times when I hit those places where I just cannot seem to break through. When that happens and I know I've checked myself against all the issues we've already discussed in this chapter, I know I need to do a temporary adjustment to my life style to regain my momentum. For a short period (measured usually in days) I will put myself on a very strict low carb diet, limited to the minimum number of carbs that can't be avoided (usually around 6 or 7 a day) and limit my daily caloric intake to a low level (for me that is usually around 1200 calories). The combination of the extremely low carbs and calories produces a high impact "charge" to my metabolism that helps me break through. I never do this for more than just a few days, and I am in good health. If that doesn't apply to you, be careful and if there are questions, check with your weight loss physician.

Regarding activities, one of the fallacies I have discovered in the "conventional wisdom" of weight loss is that "increasing activities" is often associated with what I call "islands of exercise" in an otherwise sedentary lifestyle. I would get serious about losing weight, decide to change, and start going to the gym or commit to walking 10,000 steps a day (or some other time limited exercise regimen which were essentially a break in my otherwise "normal" day). And I can't tell you how many of my patients do the same thing.

Don't get me wrong. Exercise is good, but for those of us who are starting this process out with a BMI of 35 or more, that strategy of "going to the gym" may actually work against you. What often happens is that the body sees those "islands of exercise" as something that needs to be "adjusted to" - in other words, the body actually reduces the metabolic rate to conserve fat storage to compensate for the periods of high activity. For me, not only did weight loss stop during those periods, but often with no change in what I was eating, I actually started to regain weight.

What is needed is a more balanced, level increase in activity throughout the day. That last part is the key. If the body sees the increase in activity as a fundamental change in "lifestyle" as opposed to intense periods of activity in an otherwise unchanged lifestyle, the body doesn't feel the need to adjust metabolism to store more fat...it sees the need to adjust metabolism to burn more fat.

One of my strategies is to commit to doing 5 pushups between appointments. I see enough patients every hour that I'm doing a significant number of pushups spaced out over each hour and the entire day. My body sees this as an overall increase in activity, not sporadic. And this consistently helps me to overcome sluggish weight loss.

8

EATING OUT
on the HLFC lifestyle

If you've decided you'd like to explore the High Fat Low Carb lifestyle, one of the first things you'll run into after the thrill of eating cheese omelettes and bacon for breakfast, McDonald's Double Cheeseburgers (plain, without the bun), and steak and broccoli with loads of butter for dinner wears off, is how to weed out those pesky carbs and still have some variety in your "food life."

This is especially true when it comes to eating between meals. While you'll find that desire largely disappears with the HFLC lifestyle, there are social situations where "noshing" is more or less required. And suddenly the Triscuit crowd is looking at you askance and askew as you eschew the hor d'oeuvres (See what I did there grammatically?).

And then there is the whole eating out thing. You'll quickly find restaurants have a bias toward carbohydrates and either mix them with fat (the worst combination) or go low fat high carb all the way.

In this chapter we're going to offer some helps for weathering those situations.

HIGHER END RESTAURANT STRATEGIES

OK, you're pretty creative so you'll figure out the double cheeseburger thing (also works for a Sausage McMuffin without the muffin). You'll also find you'll be going to the salad with some sort of protein on top and straight olive oil for dressing in the higher class places.

The main problem with eating out,

Social Pressure
No one likes social pressure, but it is there nonetheless. And this is especially true with the HFLC lifestyle because of the emphasis on eating the majority of your calories from fat.

Society has become so brainwashed into thinking fat is bad, even if you tell people you are on an HFLC diet, it really doesn't register with them that you are eating so much fat.

So when you eat in front of unbelievers, even though you've told them, they are still shocked (and judgmental) that you are eating so much fat. Clearly you are going to die. And probably at this meal.

though, is that there is a tendency to end up eating too much protein in relationship to the fat. Why?

Well, two reasons for that. The first is because restaurants don't tend to serve a lot of fat. Ask for a side of butter with your steak or salmon, and you'll get a couple of pats in a little silver cup. That's not nearly enough to cover the 8 oz. of protein on your plate, so your choice is to take some of the protein home (yes, real men do get doggie bags) or ask for more butter, or olive oil, or a side of mayonnaise and risk the inevitable judgment from the server.

The other reason is you run the risk of getting that same judgmental vibe from your dinner companions.

Both end up tending to influence you away from asking for enough fat to balance the protein.

And if you bull through and ask for the "side of fat" along with some "extra fat", you know you're going to end up having to explain the whole deal to your dinner companions. And that ranks right up there with vegans explaining why they're vegans. Annoying.

Our advice: go with whatever you feel comfortable asking for from the server and stop eating the protein when you can no longer balance it with fat.

Some supplemental strategies: order coffee (or decaf at night) and ask the server to get some "real cream" from the kitchen. Servers love that because it is an extra service that will likely bump up the tip. And your friends will just think you have discerning taste buds.

And if you order some coffee before and after the meal, both with real cream, you've increased your fat intake on both ends.

Another strategy is to ask for extra

When you absolutely can't avoid too many carbs

We've all been there. You're invited to a friend's house for dinner, you're thinking you can "eat around" the carbs, and BOOM! they serve you a main course of baked ziti, a side of corn, and home made chocolate cake for desert. The butter is fake, there's no reasonable place to add mayonnaise, and the amount of "counter balancing" olive oil you'd have to eat on your salad with candied pecans and raisins would float a boat.

What do you do?

Two things:

1. Eat small portions and don't be afraid to leave some on your plate.
2. Work in as much fat as you can (ask for the ziti from the part where it looks like there's the most cheese)

By limiting portion size and eating maximum available fat, you'll slow down carb absorption and give your body its best chance to "spread the carbs out".

butter when the bread comes. "Oh, that's not going to be enough butter. Can we have some more?"

Of course you aren't going to be eating the bread, but you can slide a couple or three pats of the extra butter on to your bread plate for later in the meal.

Finally, look for an appetizer that is mostly fat. More and more you see "artisan cheese plates", sometimes even as a desert. Bonus! Just watch out here, though. Cheeses are part protein and part fat, so you aren't getting the edge on your main course you would with butter, mayonnaise, or olive oil. But cheese does provide a little bump.

And stay away from dessert.

But look, let's be honest. There are times where you are going to be looking at dessert. And despite your best intentions, you're going to be forced to partake (like maybe you're with a client, you know?).

If it is available, order cheesecake. Yes, it is loaded with carbs, but it also has a ton of fat, which in this case, will likely slow the digestion of the carbs down enough that they won't have the same impact on your metabolism.

We are not giving you a bye on this. Don't think we're saying to go ahead and order cheesecake regularly. Nope. Stay away from restaurant desserts. Period. But in those rare times when you can't (not "don't want to" but really "can't") defer on dessert, go with the plain cheesecake. And order a cup of decaf with extra "real cream." And don't eat it all.

LOWER END RESTAURANT STRATEGIES

Eating out is not for wimps
Man, you'd think eating out would be a breeze, but its not. We do the HFLC diet and we prefer eating in because it is much easier to control your carb/protein/fat balance when you're doing the shopping and cooking.

At some point, you have to "man up" and not be afraid or embarrassed to ask for what you want when you eat out.

And don't feel like you have to explain it to everyone. A simple "I'm on a special diet" while not strictly true, is often more than sufficient to get through the stunned silence when you order extra butter but aren't eating bread.

Pizza restaurants are golden. Order the pizza with extra cheese, no sauce, and whatever toppings you want. Then use your fork to eat the cheese and toppings. Admit it, that's what you always wanted to do as a kid. Go for it.

Fast food is so obvious we aren't going to even deal with it here. Stay away from the bun and the condiments and any protein that is breaded. Nuff said.

Chinese and other oriental food servers present a unique issue because sugar and honey are such a critical component of their cooking. Mongolian barbecue or Moo Shoo Pork have a number of ingredients that are very high in cheap carbs. Even some of the appetizers which don't come in a sauce are often marinated in something with a lot of sugar or honey.

We've really got nothing for you here. You're going to end up eating some significant carbs, and there's not much you can do to tailor your ordering. And they typically don't serve butter or mayonnaise. Your only hope is if they have a salad option which you can add some protein on top of and slather on the olive oil. Sorry, dude.

Italian food is pretty straight forward, but still problematic. You've got to stay away from pasta. Meatballs sound good but they are often up to 50% breading. Then you've got the "parms": chicken parm, etc. The problem here is the breading which gets cemented in place by the melted cheese. And the sauce.

Best bet here is the salad route. Our key strategy is the Antipasto! It usually comes with a reasonable amount of protein and your own personal cruet of olive oil. Order it for the meal.

Record what you eat
We know we sound like a broken record on this, but we know first hand how easy it is to just "go with the flow" while you're on the road. You're tired, you're away from home, and you're hungry. You want easy. You want quick. We get it. Been there, done that, got the T-shirt.

All the more reason to make sure you log what you eat. You have to be accountable to yourself, and that silly little smart phone app is the tool to make you stop and think about the choices you are making.

As long as your eating record stays in your head, you are more likely to ignore your conscience. But when it is on your phone and computer, well, there it is. A record of your choices.

C'mon, man.

EATING ON THE ROAD

Are you a road warrior? Do you travel on business? If so, you have a number of issues that are unique to that whole process. You'd think it would be easy, given the usual assortment of choices that come with being "out and about," but nope. There are three main issues you'll run into. One is lack of choices. Two is portion sizes. Three is often a time constraint.

It's counter-intuitive but there is a real lack of choices in airports and hotels. If you are consciously trying to keep carbs out of your diet and keep your fat intake higher than your protein, the number of options available to you are severely limited.

Generally speaking most options on the road are either high carbs, low protein, low fat (think pasta or veggie options) or they are high carbs, high protein, high fat (think burgers, tacos, fried foods, etc.)

It is true that as the research continues to come in about the benefits of a HFLC lifestyle and more and more people are adopting it, there are a growing number of menu options available to travelers. If you can find them, great. But what about when you can't.

Trying to find a meal option that fits with the minimum ideal ratio of roughly equal grams of fat to grams of protein plus carbs is often difficult.

To the extent possible, use the strategies we offered with various restaurants.

PRO TIP: One of the real weapons for staying in balance, fat to carb/protein, is the individual serving of mayonnaise. You know, that rectangular package of mayo you can get at most of the fast food booths at an airport.

One of those is roughly equal to a tablespoon and a half of mayonnaise which

Pork Rinds
God's gift to a HFLC diet. They are crunchy, tasty, and about right in macronutrient balance. We don't spend any time talking about them because they are pretty much an add on food. And they don't really help rein in a runaway appetite. But they are good. And they are very low carb.

provides you with 18 grams of fat, no carbs and no protein. We always grab a handful of those suckers and jam them in our briefcase and jacket pocket.

The nice thing about them is that they last forever and you can eat one fairly surreptitiously while standing off to the side at a gate or in the back seat of a taxi. It is an immediate bolus of fat that will help to balance out any excess protein or slow down the digestion of any unwanted but unavoidable carbs you've eaten.

[Recently we've found a website that offers products designed at least partly with the road warrior in mind – and some of us stay at home types, too. Check out Adapt Your Life. This is a product line designed with the HLFC diet we're describing in mind. It isn't ours (darn it!) but we can recommend you check it out at www.adaptyourlife.com]

PRO TIP #2: Repeat after me, "bacon jerky". Yup. It's real. The HFLC lifestyle's favorite food of all time. You can find it in a number of different places including convenience stores and truck stops. We've also started to see pepperoni jerky and little links of breakfast type sausage as jerky. These are great, too.

Whenever and wherever you do find it, we recommend picking up 4 or 5 packages at a minimum. Like the mayo packets, it's jerky, so it's going to last. Put some in your briefcase, the glove compartment of your car, your gym bag, etc. It is a great meal replacement when you can't get a meal due to travel.

One downside is that, unlike the mayo, it isn't going to act as a meal supplement to balance anything out. The bacon jerky itself is an HFLC balanced food with roughly equivalent grams of fat and protein with zero carbs. So don't use it to

Please be aware that just because the package says "Lo Carb" does not mean it is really good for a high fat, low carb diet.

A couple of pointers:

1. Oft times food manufacturers make food low carb by reducing the serving size. That doesn't have any impact on the number of carbs in the package. So you need to look at the nutrition label, figure out if you're going to eat the whole package, and if you are, multiply the number of carbs by the number of servings in the package. Not so "lo carb" now, is it?

2. "Lo carb" can also be a relative term. This particular brand of this product might be lower in carbs than the competition. Cool. But you only care if the number of carbs isn't going to put you over the edge. Read the label, dude.

counteract eating too much protein or slow down the digestion of too many carbs. As we said, it's a meal replacement.

What about regular jerky? Well, be careful there, sport. It is often thought of as a HFLC choice. And maybe back a decade ago it was. But today, sugar has crept in so carbs are an issue. And in a strange attempt to emulate a "health food" you may find that many brands are also low fat. So that's probably not going to be a great choice. Although I have to admit, in a pinch, when I couldn't find bacon jerky, I ate a low carb version of beef jerky with a mayo packet or two as a meal supplement. [All the nutritionists just went into spasms when they read that, I'm sure.]

Airport convenience stores offer bags of nuts. OK. Nuts are good, but be aware of the carbs that will sneak in.

For the most part, there is enough fat in a bag of nuts to slow down the impact of the carbs. So proceed, but with caution.

Don't eat the whole bag. And don't pick the nut combinations with dried fruit or raisins. You're just eating too many carbs.

What about low carb nutritional bars?

OK. Atkins and a number of other brands put out a low carb snack or meal replacement marketed for us HFLC folks. And, label-wise, they seem to fit the profile for our lifestyle.

They're OK with a couple of caveats.

First, if you are going to eat one, eat it as a meal replacement and not a meal supplement - even if it says "snack" on the label. You are adding calories and some carbs into your meal if you use it as a supplement and you really aren't balancing out anything when you do that.

Second, only eat one a day. And maybe not one every day. They contain either a

Killer Sweet Tooth
When you eat sweets,
even low carb sweets, it
triggers a desire for more
sweets. And that can kill
your lifestyle.

Our experience is that if
you can resist eating
anything sweet (including
avoiding a safe sweetener
in your coffee) for three
days, you've probably
broken the back of your
sugar cravings.

sugar substitute or a sugar alcohol for sweetness. It's true that these do not threaten ketosis, but they do create a psychological craving for sweetness that makes it increasingly hard to resist eating something sweet the further you go down that path.

PRO TIP #3: In general, if you can stay away from things that are sweet, even if they are "safe sweet", you'll find that it is easier and easier to pass all sweets up as time goes by. We speak from experience here.

You know that sugar alcohols have a "laxative effect" right? Eating one in a day, you are probably safe. Probably. More than one, not so much. While traveling I can think of no better reason to avoid those bars that contain sugar alcohols than that.

By now you've probably realized the value of drinking your coffee with heavy cream. But it is almost impossible to get heavy cream on the road. Most restaurants and fast food places serve "half & half". That's better than milk or non-dairy creamers (which just add carbs). Half and half provides roughly 3 grams of fat and 1 gram of protein and carbohydrates each per ounce (two "dollops" in your coffee).

Obviously the best is heavy cream. Starbucks offers heavy cream, if you request it by name. Dunkin' Donuts uses light cream, which is about half way between half and half and heavy cream. I search those franchises out.

So adding cream of any variety to your coffee is a great way to balance out on the road.

Elsewhere we've talked about the value of using a smartphone based app to track your nutritional intake. We've talked about how important it is to keep track of what you are putting in your mouth, rather than relying on your memory. Nowhere is that more important than when you are on the road. Get the app. Do the discipline.

9

EATING IN
recipes for the
HLFC lifestyle

One of the great things about the HFLC lifestyle is how creative you can get with the fundamentals. Creating interesting and delicious dishes is very easy because the high fat of the HFLC allows you to use very rich ingredients with tons of flavor.

Over the years we've collected some of our favorites to share with you. Like all things HFLC, these are loaded with flavor and very satisfying so you won't have to eat a regular size portion to feel full and content.

In the following recipes we've focused on deserts and snacks because these are typically the hardest to find "store bought". There are a number of "Low Carb" recipe books on the market for main and side dishes. Just be aware when you buy one, it is probably skewed to the "low fat" version of "low carb" so you'll need to adjust the recipe to get to the balance of fat, protein, and carbs you want.

Enjoy!

No Carb Individual Pan Pizza or Taco Shell
Ingredients:
1C Shredded mozzarella or other cheese
1T Olive oil (optional)
Toppings of your choice (omit if you are making a taco shell)

Tools:
Non-stick omelette or small fry pan
Spatula

Preparation:
If the pan is truly non-stick, you won't need the olive oil. But if it is older and tends to stick, add the olive oil and put the pan on the stove to begin to heat up

Pizza Method:
Cover the bottom of the pan with a layer of shredded cheese

Add the topping(s) of your choice - simple is better

Cover with a thin layer of cheese to tie the toppings in

Sauté at a medium high heat until the cheese in the middle of the top is starting to melt

Remove to cutting board, allow a minute or two for the cheese to bind, cut into six pieces

Taco Shell Method

Cover the bottom of the pan with the shredded cheese

Sauté at a medium high heat until the cheese in the middle of the top is starting to melt

Remove to cutting board and quickly roll into the shape of a taco shell and allow to cool

Fill with toppings and eat

Notes:

Too many toppings and the cheese on the top doesn't melt and the whole thing falls apart when you slice it.

The cheese on the bottom is going to burn. You want it to burn because it is going to cool to be the crust.

Do not cook at too high a heat. Medium high is usually enough to get a crisp crusty bottom but give time for the rest of the cheese to melt. If in doubt, turn the heat down a bit.

If you can't imagine a pizza without sauce, add some diced tomatoes before the other toppings. Don't add any juice, just the meat of the tomatoes. It will add carbs, but you've got plenty to spare on this meal.

TACO: note that your shell will be superior to the standard flour or corn meal variety because it won't get soggy. But also note that if your ingredients are wet, since they are not being absorbed by the shell, they will run out the ends. Be prepared. Also be prepared for everyone else to want one of your taco shells.

Low Carb Protein Shake Meal Replacement

Ingredients:

1 scoop Isopure (or similar whey protein isolate)

6T Heavy Cream

5oz Water

1T Chia seeds (optional)

Method:

Place powder and chia seeds (if used) in an extra large glass or plastic cup

Add cream and water

Mix thoroughly with an immersion blender and drink

Notes
The chia seeds are for extra non-soluble fiber to keep you "moving". We use them typically once a day with consistent results. They don't add any flavor to the shake, and you will inevitably leave some in the glass, but that's fine.

Nutritional Info:
Calories 412 for the shake, 60 for the chia
Fat 33g
Protein 12.5g
Fiber 5g
Net Carbs 0.5g

These values are for illustration. They will change depending on the type of shake mix you use, although not a lot. While we use the Isopure Low and No carb flavors, there are others that are good. But even within the Isopure brand, the nutritional values fluctuate from flavor to flavor. Also, the calories seem a lot, but remember these are mostly coming from fat, and your body will use those calories for a long lasting energy source all morning or afternoon long.

Flourless Chocolate Cake w/ Optional Berry Sauce
Ingredients:
8oz. unsweetened baking chocolate
1 stick real butter
1C Splenda
4 large eggs

Tools:
Double boiler or two pans that can be rigged like one (see notes)
8" round cake pan
Cooking parchment
Hand held mixer
Instant read thermometer

Preparation:
* Preheat oven to 325
* Line the cake pan with the parchment, up the sides
* Lightly coat the parchment with butter/Pam/oil

Method:

1. Break the baking chocolate into small chunks and heat on the stovetop using a double boiler until melted and smooth. While the chocolate is melting…

2. Melt the butter in a separate pan being careful not to burn it

3. Turn off the heat under the butter and mix in the Splenda

4. Separate the eggs, yolks in one bowl, whites in another.

5. Beat the yolks on high until thick and blend in the Splenda mixture. Then, very slowly, stir in the butter by hand being careful to do it small enough amounts so you are not cooking the yolks.

6. Beat the whites until fluffy and they can hold peaks. (best in a chilled bowl with chilled beaters)

7. Fold the melted chocolate into the butter/Splenda/yolk mixture slowly, no more than 1/3 at a time. As you add the chocolate, stir just long enough so that the streaks disappear, then add more chocolate.

8. Once the yolk mixture and chocolate are completely mixed, very slowly blend in the egg whites, again stirring only enough to make the streaks disappear.

9. Transfer the entire mixture into a prepared cake pan and place on the center rack of the oven.

10. Bake at 325 for about 10 minutes.

11. Check the temperature at the center with an instant read thermometer. Continue to check every five minutes or so and remove when the center is 150 degrees.

12. Allow to cool for about 10 minutes, remove from pan but leave the parchment in place, cover, refrigerate for a minimum of 2 hours…overnight is best.

13. Slice into 8 pieces

Notes:

- A double boiler is ideal but you can fake one by either using two pots, one which fits into another and which fairly tightly seals around the sides, or a pot and a glass or ceramic mixing bowl (that is not temperature sensitive) that the same tight seal. The trick is that you do not want a lot of steam to escape while the bottom pot is boiling because if it does, and it condenses in the chocolate, the chocolate is ruined.

- If you do not have cooking parchment, DO NOT use wax paper or aluminum foil in its place. Just coat the cake pan with oil and flour making sure all the surfaces are well prepared.

- The "optional berry sauce" can be prepared as needed. I recommend it because the cake can often be very dry in spite of the fact it has no flour. In a sauce pan, heat up a jigger of vodka (chocolate or coffee flavored vodka works well, by the way) per serving. Add to the heating vodka, both raspberries and blackberries in equal amounts, about a half cup of each per serving, and allow the vodka to come to a boil. While stirring the mixture you will note that the raspberries will break down and thicken and color the vodka, and the blackberries will remain whole but begin to turn reddish in color. At that point your mixture is done. The alcohol will have boiled off and you will be left with a wonderful "slurry" of berries which can be used as a topping for the cake. I recommend reheating the cake while the berry sauce is cooking, and serving the whole mixture in a shallow soup bowl or a plate with steeper sides. If you have Newberg dishes (like they use in restaurants for broiled scallops etc.) those are ideal and the cake can be reheated right in those.

- In lieu of the berry sauce, melted butter makes a decadent topping.

Near Zero Carb Flax Bread
An ideal, high density, almost zero carb, gluten free quick bread. It is high in calories relative to other breads and so traditional dieters should beware. However for those who are not on calorie restricted diets, especially those on HFLC diets (High Fat Low Carb), this bread is a nice addition.

Ingredients:
Dry:
2C flax seed flour or meal (can substitute Almond Flour - add 3T of Xanthan Gum)
1T baking powder
1t salt
3 packets Stevia

Wet:
4 whole eggs
5T olive oil (the lightest flavor possible)
1/2c water
1/4t vanilla extract

Directions:
1. Preheat oven to 350 degrees
2. Coat a small loaf pan with whatever type of oil used above
3. Mix all dry ingredients
4. Whisk all wet ingredients
5. Add together and whisk
6. Scrape into loaf pan and shake to even out

7. Bake at 350 for about 25-30 minutes (test with dry toothpick in the center)

Notes:
This recipe can also be made into muffins: divide batter into muffin pans and reduce baking time to about 10-15 minutes.

You can substitute 2 whole eggs and 5 egg whites for the 4 whole eggs to reduce calories.

Instead of olive oil, you can use coconut or flax oil but it will affect the flavor of the bread.

The vanilla extract is a flavor "mask" for the stronger flax flavor. It can be omitted if desired.

You can start with whole flax seeds and use a food processor to grind them into flour. Start with more than 2 cups of seeds as you will need two cups of the finished product.

Commentary:
The net impact carbs (total carbs minus fiber) is .5g per slice. Normally a bread this low in carbs either has the consistency or card board or the taste thereof. After trying numerous recipes, I settled on this one, which is a tweak of a fairly common flax bread recipe. Don't vary the recipe with the first loaf. Do it according to what I've done below. The second loaf you can start futzing with the recipe so you know if you are improving it or not.

Three important things… use dark flax seed meal/flour if at all possible. That seems to have a more benign flavor. And use olive oil that is light/mild in flavor. The first time I made this, I used light flax and a fairly robust olive oil. The two combined to produce an almost fishy type of flavor. Third, try it with the whole eggs first. The extra yolks also tend to mollify the flavor of the flax.

You can substitute almond flour and add a little xanthan gum to help with texture. The almond flour is higher in both carbs and calories than flax, but this is made up for by the fact you can get more slices out of a loaf. So you get a lighter, better tasting bread that is slightly fewer calories for the extra 2 g. of carbs per slice.

One last point: you almost can't over bake this bread. It is almost cake-like when done with all the eggs in it. Test for doneness in the very center of the loaf and make sure the toothpick comes out dry, otherwise you'll find you have a very nice bread, with a "cream" center.

Nutrition info - flax:
(1 serving = 1 slice, 14 slices per loaf)
192 cal
  17 g fat
   7 g carbs
   6.5 g fiber
   4 g protein

Nutrition info - almond:
(1 serving = 1 slice, 16 slices per loaf)
176 cal
  17 g fat
   5 g carbs
   2.5 g fiber
   6 g protein

Near Zero Carb Flax Crackers

Ingredients:
¼ C whole flax seeds
¾ C flax meal/flour
2 Eggs
1 T grated Parmesan, Romano, or other hard grating cheese
1 t caraway seeds (or dill or sage or rosemary or garlic, etc.)
Salt (preferably coarse ground)

Method:
Preheat the oven to 325 degrees
Mix all the ingredients except the salt in a mixing bowl
Let the mixture stand for about 10 minutes while preparing a cookie sheet
Roll out the mixture (between parchment or waxed paper is helpful) to the thickness of a wheat thin
Using a cookie cutter or butter knife cut the dough into pieces roughly about the size of a wheat thin
Place on the prepared cookie sheet and add salt to taste
Bake for 10 minutes, turn, and bake the second side for another 3-5 minutes depending on the amount of crispiness desired - being careful not to burn
Remove and allow to fully cool before storing

Makes about 50 +- crackers

Nutritional Information:

Serving size: 10 Crackers
Calories - 409
Fat - 32g
Carbohydrates - 20g
Fiber - 18g
   Net Carbs - 2g
Protein - 14g

Buttered Salted Pecans

You are going to love this. I had been looking for a good snack that could double as a sort of hor d'oeuvres when we have folks over for an adult beverage. Nuts are the obvious choice but the amount of almonds or cashews you eat often makes me overly carb conscious. Then I found pecans. They are never in the snack nut section at the store so I never thought about them. But I was in the baking aisle and noticed them there…uncooked. So I bought a bag, threw them in a large frying pan with a stick of butter, sautéd them until they were crispy (and some of them looked a little burnt), and then drained and salted them. Man oh man, everybody loves them. And it is right in the HFLC "zone".

Ingredients:
1 bag of pecans (16 oz.)
1 stick of butter (Kerrygold is great if you can find it)
Coarse ground sea salt

Method:
Melt the butter over medium heat
Add pecans
Stir almost continuously being careful to lift nuts up from the bottom to the top
Remove from heat when 10% of the nuts appear burnt and the rest are crispy (The burnt ones have great flavor, by the way)
Allow to drain in a large bowl lined with paper towels
Cool or can be served warm
Store leftovers in the refrigerator

Nutritional information:
Serving size: about 15 halves (roughly a handful)
235 calories
25.4g fat
1.2 net carbs
2.7g protein

That's a 90/10 ratio of fat to protein/carbs.

Zero Carb Chia Crackers

Ingredients:
1 C Chia seeds
2 Eggs
1 T grated Parmesan, Romano, or other hard grating cheese
1 t caraway seeds (or dill or sage or rosemary or garlic, etc.)
Salt (preferably coarse ground)

Method:
Preheat the oven to 325 degrees
Mix all the ingredients except the salt in a mixing bowl
Let the mixture stand for about 10 minutes while preparing a cookie sheet
Use a large wooden spoon or spatula to flatten the mixture on parchment paper is to the thickness of a Trisket - do not separate the individual crackers yet
Using a cookie cutter, pizza cutter, or butter knife score the dough into roughly the size of a Trisket.
Place the parchment on the cookie sheet and add salt to taste
Bake for 20 minutes, turn, separate, and bake the second side for another 20 minutes depending on the amount of crispiness desired - being careful not to burn
Remove and allow to fully cool before storing

Makes about 30 +- crackers

Nutritional Information:
Serving size: 10 Crackers
Calories - 403
Fat - 22g
Carbohydrates - 27g
Fiber - 27g
  Net Carbs - 0g
Protein - 19g

Chia has a "fishy" flavor so you will definitely need a flavoring like caraway that has a strong enough flavor to "carry" the cracker. Otherwise you'll eat them with cheese or a dip but not plain.

Near Zero Carb Ice Cream Custard – Plain Old Vanilla

(Old fashioned ice cream, rich with the flavor of vanilla and custard)

Ingredients:
3 cups of heavy cream
1 cup of water
1 cup of Splenda
2 tablespoons of vanilla extract
5 large egg yolks

Method:
Mix together all the ingredients in a large mixing bowl until thoroughly blended

Transfer the mixture to a large sauce pan and heat while stirring, being careful to NOT allow the mixture to come to a boil – when you see it start to steam, take it off the heat.

Transfer the mixture back into the bowl, cover, and refrigerate overnight.

Use your ice cream maker and follow manufacturer's instructions.

Store in the freezer in individual serving size containers for the best tasting ice cream custard ever.

NOTE: you can add flavorings to the mixture or berries to the ice cream process, but honestly the flavor of the vanilla is so rich you will find you don't need it.

Nutritional information for a 5 oz serving
291 cal
  28.6 g fat
   0.3 g carbs
   0 g fiber
   1.1 g protein

Near Zero Carb Ice Cream – Plain Old Vanilla

This is for those who don't like/want the custard like flavor of the previous recipe.

Ingredients:
2 cups heavy cream
1 cup of water
1 cup of Splenda
1 tablespoon of vanilla

Method:
Combine the ingredients, stir thoroughly, and refrigerate for at least 2

hours.

You'll need an ice cream maker to do this. Follow the particular directions for your brand. When done, it can be eaten right away as soft serve, or put into smaller containers and frozen for a "hard serve" consistency.

Notes:

Do NOT store the finished product in one container. It will be impossible to get a single serving out. You'll need to store it in individual serving size containers.

When removing it from the freezer you will need to let it sit for about 15-20 minutes until it gets soft enough to spoon.

For flavored ice cream you can add the following ingredients:

Chocolate: Unsweetened baking cocoa

Strawberry or other berry flavors: Cut up 5 or 6 medium size strawberries into very small pieces and add during the ice cream making process about half way through

Pistachio – add a teaspoon of almond extract during the mixing phase and about a cup of shelled pistachios, not too finely chopped about half way through the ice cream making process.

Nutritional information per 5 oz serving for vanilla flavored
202 cal
  20 g fat
    0.1 g carbs
    0 g fiber
    0 g protein

Zero Carb Quick Ice Cream

A no muss, no fuss version for those of you who are too impatient to wait overnight for your ice cream.

Ingredients:
1 cup water
1 cup heavy cream
1 pkg sugar free flavored jello

Method:

Bring water to a boil and stir in flavored gelatin packet. Stir the gelatin while boiling for 30-60 seconds or until completely dissolved.

Add the cream to the hot mixture and stir in thoroughly

Refrigerate the mixture for two hours

You can eat it as a creamy jello or you can separate the mixture into smaller containers and put in the freezer for about one hour before eating.

Nutritional information for a 5 oz serving
104 cal
   10 g fat
    0 g carbs
    0 g fiber
    0.4 g protein

Near Zero Carb Chocolate
Ingredients:
2 cups cocoa powder
3/4 cup butter, softened to room temperature
3/4 cup Splenda
2/3 cup heavy cream, room temperature
1/4 teaspoon salt
1 cup water

Instructions
Heat the water in a medium-sized saucepan until simmering.

Cream the cocoa powder and butter together into a paste.

Add the cocoa mixture to the hot water. Bring it back to simmering, and then remove from heat and transfer the cocoa mixture to a bowl.

Sift the Splenda and salt together in a separate bowl to eliminate any lumps.

Add to the cocoa mixture and stir well to combine.

Add the cream slowly and stir.

Pour the chocolate mixture in thin layers into molds and freeze or refrigerate until firm.

The recipe doesn't produce tempered chocolate, it is a more firm truffle consistency. You can make it harder by substituting softened cocoa butter for dairy butter - that will give it a raw chocolate consistency (firmer than truffles, but softer than a candy bar). If you want it harder still, you can reduce the amount of water or eliminate it all together using a double boiler to heat the cocoa mixture instead. The thinner you pour it, the harder it will become as well; thick chocolate molds will produce a fudgier consistency.

About the Authors

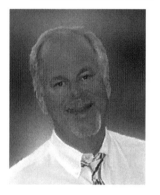

SKIP SIMONDS

William W. "Skip" Simonds is a semi-retired businessman, consultant, and lay minister.

In addition, Skip is involved in community leadership and church activities in the small island community where he lives in Maine.

As he "glides" into retirement, Skip has continued his lifelong love of writing by authoring a number of different articles and books. Among them are The Motive Gifts, Get Over It (how to get to forgiveness that sticks), and The Measure of a Man. The latter is based on his popular "King/Warrior/Sage/Lover" work with men helping them reach their full potential. In addition he is the leader of numerous King/Warrior/Sage/Lover seminars and workshops for men that have been conducted internationally.

Skip has collaborated on this book with his nephew, Dr. Simonds, due to the phenomenal weight loss he experienced as a result of working with Dr. Simonds. Wickham's "no BS" approach to diet, along with the clarity of understanding he imparted paired with Skip's love of writing, suggested the collaboration for this book.

Skip has an advanced degree in psychology and does counseling through LifeFlow, a Christian ministry he has founded. Skip and his wife, Betsey, live on the coast of Maine and share a passion for music and singing. And Skip, like his nephew, is an avid golfer (when the Maine weather permits).

WICKHAM B. SIMONDS, M.D.

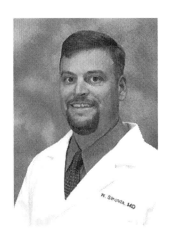

Dr. Simonds is the founder of Dr. Simonds Weight Loss and currently practices Obesity Medicine with offices in Durham and Raleigh. Dr. Simonds is board certified by the American Board of Emergency Medicine and the American Board of Obesity Medicine. He was Chief Resident during his residency in Emergency Medicine at Penn State University/York Hospital. Dr. Simonds received his MD from East Carolina University after graduating Summa Cum Laude with a BS in Biology from Campbell University. He is a member of the American Society of Bariatric Physicians and The Obesity Society.

He was raised in Durham, N.C. and graduated high school from Cresset Christian Academy in Durham. He has served his country in the U.S. Army with duty stations in Korea, Louisiana, and Iraq. The latter involved deployments in (1)1990 and 1991 for Operation Desert Shield and Storm, (2) 2003 to Southern Iraq in support of Operation Enduring and Iraqi Freedom, and (3) 2005 to Iraq in support of Operation Iraqi Freedom.

Dr. Simonds is married to his wife Anna who is a Registered Nurse. They have four children and two grandchildren. He is active in church and community activities in addition to being an avid golfer.

Printed in Great Britain
by Amazon